Drug Therapy in Rheumatology Nursing

Edited by

SARAH RYAN BSc MSc RGN

Clinical Nurse Specialist Rheumatology

W

WHURR PUBLISHERS

LONDON

© 1999 Whurr Publishers
First published 1999 by
Whurr Publishers Ltd
19b Compton Terrace, London N1 2UN, England

British Library Cataloguing in Publication Data
A catalogue record for this book is available from the British
Library.

ISBN: 186156 114 8

Printed and bound in the UK by Athenaeum Press Ltd,
Gateshead, Tyne & Wear

Contents

Contributors

Ann Brownfield BSc (Hons) RGN, Ward Sister, Haywood Hospital, Burslem, Stoke on Trent

Janet Cushnaghan MSc MCSP, Rheumatology Clinical Specialist, Rheumatology Department, Hereford County Hospital, Hereford

Jackie Hill MPhil RGN FRCN, Rheumatology Nurse Practitioner, Clinical Pharmacology Unit, Chapel Allerton Hospital, Leeds

Jacqueline McDowell BSc(Hons) RGN, National Certificate District Nursing, Clinical Nurse Specialist, Rheumatology Department, Hereford County Hospital, Hereford

Sarah Ryan BSc(Hons) MSc RGN, Clinical Nurse Specialist Rheumatology, Haywood Hospital, Burslem, Stoke on Trent

Margaret Ann Voyce SRN, Rheumatology Nurse Practitioner, Rheumatology Department, Royal Cornwall Hospital (City), Truro, Cornwall

Preface

This text provides a comprehensive exploration on the drug treatment utilised in the management of rheumatological and related conditions. It will provide a valuable resource to all nurses and other health care professionals in the care of patients with a rheumatological complaint, be it in the hospital, community or research setting.

The philosophy of this book is based on a patient-focused approach to care, enabling the patient to become an active participant and not a passive recipient of care management. Non-compliancy in patients with rheumatoid arthritis can range from 38% to 78% (Bradley LA, Adherence with treatment regimens among adult rheumatoid arthritis patients: current status and future directions. Arthritis Care and Research 1989;2: s33–39). This may well be attributed to an lack of prior understanding of the purpose of the drug therapy, and it is therefore essential that the nurse ascertains the patient's perceptions and expectations before the commencement of any new therapy.

Patients will often require a combination of drug therapy to provide symptomatic control and disease suppression. The addition or alteration to a patient's drug treatment will require exploration of the patient's (and their family's) expectations to ensure that all treatment has meaning and relevance within the patient's contextual framework.

The book contains five parts, each divided into several short chapters; each part begins with learning objectives which will guide the reader as to the contents of the following chapters. The book is based on clinical and research findings, to enable the adoption of evidence-based practice within care settings.

The parts of the book progress in a logical manner, providing information on:

- rheumatological conditions
- the classification, function, action and side effects of pharmaceutical agents
- the role of the nurse in drug therapy
- patient education
- the provision of community care.

The recurring themes of education, partnership and empowerment will be evident and integrated throughout the text.

The primary aims of this book include:

- A development of an understanding of those rheumatological conditions where drug treatment can be most effective.
- The provision of information on different disease processes, so that the utilisation of drug therapy can be placed in context.
- Increasing knowledge for nurses and other health professionals on the classification of drugs in common use, including analgesia, non-steroidal anti-inflammatory drugs (NSAIDs), drug-modifying antirheumatic agents (DMARDs), cytotoxic drugs, steroids and treatment for gout. This will incorporate the purpose of administration, potential side effects and common dosages in use.
- An exploration of the role of the nurse in the management of drug therapy, focusing on the knowledge and skills required to undertake drug surveillance and assessment of interventions.
- A comprehensive exploration of patient education: theories, principles, content and delivery of education are discussed.
- An investigation into the advancement of seamless care between the primary and secondary sectors.

This book can be used as a reference text for those nurses who seek specific answers about one mode of drug intervention, e.g. gold therapy, as well as providing in-depth information on the principles and components of a wide range of drug therapies for clinicians specialising in this field.

The nurse performs a pivotal role in guiding, supporting and educating the patient and the family to manage their condition effectively. The utilisation of this text will enable practitioners to develop and advance their practice to the benefit of the patient.

Sarah Ryan BSc MSc RGN

Part 1
Rheumatological conditions

JANET CUSHNAGHAN AND JACKIE McDOWELL

After reading the chapters in Part 1 you should be able to:

- Discuss the anatomy and physiology of the musculoskeletal system in health and illness
- Describe the process of inflammation and the immune response
- Develop an understanding of the rheumatic diseases where drug therapy is required
- Discuss the effects of rheumatic disease on physical, psychological and social well-being

1.1 Classification and features of rheumatic conditions

The primary objective of this book is to provide the nurse with the knowledge and subsequent understanding of the role drug therapy plays in the management of rheumatological conditions. It is essential therefore that the nurse must have a good knowledge and understanding of rheumatological conditions themselves.

Rheumatology is the branch of medicine dealing with disorders of the joints, muscles, tendons and ligaments. Arthritis and the rheumatic diseases in general constitute the major cause of chronic disability in the UK, where it is estimated that 20 million individuals have a rheumatic disease, of whom 6–8 million are severely affected (Weller 1997).

The terms *arthritis* and *rheumatism or rheumatic disease* encompass a host of conditions causing much pain and suffering to those affected. The burden of these diseases is felt not only by the sufferers and their families but also by the community in terms of the cost of health care and the loss of working days. Because of the diversity of rheumatic conditions, it is helpful to classify them into groups. This may be undertaken in different ways, incorporating:

* clinical and laboratory features
* disease mechanisms, e.g. autoimmunity
* anatomical structures involved
* genetic factors
* organ systems involved and specific abnormalities or deficiencies.

Classification is hampered by the absence of firm aetiological evidence for most diseases, but for this chapter we intend to use a simplified classification corresponding to the philosophy of drug therapy which is the main purpose of this text. Table 1.1 classifies the rheumatic diseases according to the presence or absence of

inflammation, and further sub-classifies inflammatory arthritis
according to associations that may be present.

Table 1.1 Classification of rheumatic diseases

Inflammatory arthritis	Rheumatoid arthritis
	Juvenile Idiopathic Arthritis (JIA)
	Polymyalgia rheumatica
Associated with spondylitis	Ankylosing spondylitis
	Reiter's syndrome
	Psoriatic arthritis
Associated with infectious agents	Septic arthritis
	Reactive arthritis
Associated with crystals	Gout
	Pseudogout
Non-inflammatory	Osteoarthritis
	Fibromyalgia
Connective tissue disorders	Systemic Lupus Erythematosus
	Scleroderma
	Polymyositis

Symptoms of rheumatic disease can be determined by clinical
history taking and thorough physical examination. Laboratory and
radiographic investigations can aid diagnosis and eliminate certain
features, but nothing can replace the clinician's clinical skills and
pattern recognition. Patients with a rheumatological condition often
experience the symptoms of pain, swelling, stiffness and loss of function. These symptoms give rise to impairments which in turn may
produce handicap or disability, depending on the interaction of environmental, resource and psychological factors. The consequences of
disease have been described in a model by the World Health Organisation (WHO 1980) as follows:

- *Impairment:* any loss or abnormality of psychological or anatomical structure or function.
- *Disability:* any restriction or lack (resulting from impairment) of
  ability to perform an activity in the manner or within the range
  considered normal for a human being.
- *Handicap:* a disadvantage for an individual resulting from impairment or disability that limits or prevents the fulfilment of a role
  that is normal (depending on age, sex and cultural factors) for
  that individual.

One of the primary objectives of the clinical history is to ascertain a greater understanding of the pain:

- is it inflammatory?
- what is the origin of its presentation?
- what are the aggravating factors?
- what is its temporal pattern?
- are there any constitutional symptoms suggesting a systemic illness, such as fever or weight loss?

Pain

Arthralgia implies pain originating from or around a joint, but not necessarily from within the joint itself. Periarticular structures may be responsible for the pain, or it may be referred from somewhere away from the joint. Pain originating from joint structures should be improved by resting the joint and aggravated by stretching the joint or weight bearing.

Stiffness

Stiffness after prolonged immobility suggests inflammatory joint disease or synovitis. Stiffness alone is a non-specific symptom and can be present in other diseases such as parkinsonism. It is also present in older individuals. Clinically significant stiffness lasts more than 30 minutes, and in inflammatory disease the duration of stiffness is proportional to the severity of inflammation.

Swelling

Swelling may be due to synovitis, cellulitis or oedema and it is important to distinguish between them. Joint swelling may be due to soft tissue swelling or synovitis or it may be due to bony swelling indicating osteoarthritis.

Joint involvement

The pattern of joint involvement, including its symmetry, is helpful in making a diagnosis, although it should be noted that there is considerable overlap between the major causes of inflammatory polyarthritis.

Function

Loss of function is an important consequence to the patient and should be assessed in work, leisure and home activities. Functional ability depends on need, motivation and environmental factors. The assessment of function is discussed later in this chapter.

Epidemiology

Epidemiology is the study of the incidence, distribution and determinants of disease in populations in order to identify causes and ultimately lead to prevention (Table 1.2). In studying the epidemiology of rheumatic disease it is important that diagnostic criteria are used to ensure standardisation of disease definition and allow comparisons between populations. Criteria which are designed for research purposes or for entry into clinical trials may not be suitable for routine clinical practice. The prevalence estimates for selected rheumatological disorders are shown in Table 1.3.

Table 1.2 Epidemiological definitions

Incidence	The number of new cases of disease per unit time (e.g. cases per annum)
Prevalence	Total number of cases of the disease at a given time point in a defined population
Morbidity	Number of cases with a defined outcome of the disease
Mortality	Number of cases dying from the disease/unit time (e.g. deaths/annum)

Table 1.3 Prevalence estimates for selected rheumatological disorders

Disorder	Estimated prevalence (%)
Arthropathies	
Rheumatoid arthritis	1.0
In children <16 years	0.06
Osteoarthritis	
Moderate/severe radiological changes in hands or feet	23.0
Knee	3.8
Hip	1.3
Inflammatory arthropathies	
Ankylosing spondylitis	0.1
Psoriatic arthropathy	0.1
Crystalline arthritis	1.0
Connective tissue disease	
Systemic Lupus Erythematosus	0.006
Systemic sclerosis	0.002
Back troubles	>20.00

Mortality from musculoskeletal disorders is low. The major impact in the population is in terms of morbidity and disability. Osteoarthritis is the most common type of arthritis and its frequency increases with age. Back complaints represent a quarter to a third of all musculoskeletal morbidity.

1.2 Anatomy and physiology of the musculoskeletal system

Before learning about the pathology of rheumatic diseases it is important to have an understanding of the anatomy and physiology of the musculoskeletal system in health. The musculoskeletal system serves several purposes:

- providing stable support
- facilitating movement
- protecting vital organs
- allowing for growth and renewal over the lifetime of the individual (Simkin 1994).

Components of the musculoskeletal system are muscle, bone, tendons, ligaments, cartilage and synovial tissue. All musculoskeletal tissues are supplied by the circulation and guided and protected by their innervation.

Muscle

Skeletal or striated muscle provides the energy or driving force for musculoskeletal activity. Chemical energy derived from foodstuffs is ultimately converted to the mechanical energy required to do work. Individual striated fibres are bundled in perimysial tissue that transmits the force of muscle contraction through tendons to attachments on bone. Each fibre can only work in the direction of its long axis and it is only through the variety of arrangements within muscles and the cooperation between muscles that allows the full range of activities possible by man.

8

Bone

No muscle contraction would be effective unless it could produce directed motion through a skeletal lever. Each effective motion comes about as muscles act on bones to move the limbs, head or torso. In some cases the mechanical advantage of the muscle is poor and it exerts substantial transarticular compressive forces in order to generate the desired movement. The bones of the skeleton have evolved to withstand and distribute these forces. Bone is characterised by the deposition of hydroxyapatite crystals in a well organised collagenous matrix. There are two types of mature bone; compact and trabecular.

- *Compact* bone is predominant and found in the shafts of long bones. The shafts of long bones contain little or no internal osseous structure, but have a marrow cavity filled with fat and loose interstitial tissue. The bone is covered by a sensitive periosteum that is capable of new bone formation.
- *Trabecular* bone refers to the cross-braced architecture found beneath articular surfaces and in the vertebral bodies. All trabeculae undergo remodelling through ongoing processes of osteoclastic resorption and osteoblastic formation of bone.

Cartilage

The contact surfaces of bones are covered by a cushion of cartilage. For the most part this is hyaline articular cartilage which is principally made up of water. Its structure is of proteoglycan aggregates restrained within a framework of type II collagen fibres. These aggregates are made up of keratan sulphate and chondroitin sulphate. Cartilage is remarkably firm and resilient. It undergoes continuous turnover, the principal players in this being the chondrocytes which are individually active but relatively sparse so the overall metabolic activity of cartilage is relatively low. Normal hyaline cartilage lacks blood vessels and nerves and relies for nutrition on adjacent structures, the synovial microvessels.

The *synovial fluid* is the vehicle carrying nutrients to the chondrocytes and returning waste products to the blood stream. The absence of nerves in articular cartilage means that damage to this structure alone cannot be painful but in conjunction with the involvement of adjacent soft tissues or subjacent bone will cause pain. A second type of cartilage is fibrocartilage, found at sites subject to shearing forces or under tensile stress. Examples include the moon-shaped cartilages called *menisci* over each tibial plateau and the principal load-bearing region in the roof of the acetabulum. This type of cartilage is more notable for its fibrous component (mainly type 1 collagen) than for its proteoglycan composition.

Synovium

The synovium is a living lining and covers all intra-articular surfaces other than the articulating areas of cartilage. Healthy synovium is a thin structure, with a normal depth of 25–35 μm. It is made up of a well-organised matrix of numerous microfibrils and abundant proteoglycan aggregates. Within this matrix lies the synovial cells. The structure has protective and synthetic capabilities.

Ligaments and tendons

- *Ligaments* are strong bundles of parallel type 1 collagen fibres that serve as 'check-reins' to prevent inappropriate movements. Each hinge joint, for example, is bordered by collateral ligaments to limit movements to flexion and extension. Every ligament runs from bone to bone.
- *Tendons* act as active drivers of joint motion as opposed to passive restrainers (ligaments).

Tendons and ligaments insert into bone at anatomic sites known as *entheses*.

Tendon sheaths and bursae

Tendons connect muscle bodies to sometimes distant insertion sites, and therefore often run through sheaths to avoid adherence to other structures. Similarly, points of potential friction such as those between ligaments, bony prominences and overlying skin are often protected by lubricating bursae. These flimsy structures are flattened sacks lined by a tissue that is histologically indistinguishable from synovium. They contain a fluid that appears synovial. It is no surprise, therefore, that tendon sheaths and bursae are the targets of the same inflammatory diseases that affect synovial joints.

Synovial joints

Synovial joints are the commonest type of articulation in the body. They are actively driven by muscles and tendons, stabilised by ligaments, cushioned by hyaline cartilage and both nourished and lubricated by synovial tissue. A film of synovial fluid lubricates the bearing surfaces and the adjacent interfaces of synovium on cartilage and synovium on synovium.

Physiology

Physiology is the study of how living things work. The principal function of almost all joints is movement. Microscopic examination of synovium and cartilage shows them to be composed of metabolically active cells. This implies that they have the same nutritional requirements as other tissues, produce similar waste products and respond to hormonal and other metabolic stimuli in ways analogous to other tissues. Joints age, as do other tissues, with subsequent effects on function. Aspects of physiology include circulation, lymphatics, pressure, diffusion, temperature and innervation. Changes in one 'system' can have clinically important effects on another, and all are uniquely modified by physical movement.

Circulation

Joints require a blood supply to ensure the health of the cartilage that lacks blood vessels of its own. The nearest available blood vessels are the capillaries of the synovium. Transport of nutrients is dependent on diffusion. The synovium and synovial space has a major role in facilitating metabolic exchange and in maintaining a normal joint space environment. Large blood vessels of the limbs pass the articular regions, and feeder vessels enter and leave the joint capsule at positions that protect them from mechanical embarrassment during movement.

Lymphatics

There is a typical lymphatic system in the synovium but not in the cartilage. Synovial lymphatics carry excess fluid, high molecular weight solutes and protein, tiny particulates and some cells out of the joint. This transfer is powered by normal movement of the joint.

Intra-articular pressure

Normal intra-articular pressure in a resting joint is sub-atmospheric. In conditions where there is an abnormal volume of fluid in the joint the pressure will rise non-linearly. The resulting pressure–volume curve defines the compliance of the joint space and its surrounding connective tissue.

Motion

Motion is the function of diarthrodial joints, but motion itself affects the physiology and health of the joint. If a joint is immobilised, cartilage thins and loses its mechanical properties. The application and release of weight-bearing forces play a part in joint lubrication and in the diffusion of substances in and out of cartilage. Joint movement is also required to maintain health by:

- maintaining normal strength and coordination of muscles
- preserving bone mass
- maintaining desired weight
- preserving normal range of joint motion
- increasing blood flow to the synovial tissues
- permitting the lymphatic system to clear the joint of particulates and excess fluid.

Innervation

There are no nerves in articular hyaline cartilage. Most of the synovium is insensitive but there are small and isolated areas that are painful when stimulated mechanically (Kellgren and Samuel 1950). Small-diameter nerve fibres are present within the confines of the capsule. The capsule, intra-articular fat pads, ligaments, periosteum, muscles and adjacent bone have abundant innervation. The major function of joint innervation appears to be proprioception – the perception of joint position, and the direction and velocity of movement.

Temperature

The normal intra-articular temperature of peripheral joints is far less than 37°C. Temperature is largely a function of blood flow. Joint movement increases joint temperature.

Anatomy and physiology in inflammatory arthrititic conditions

The inflammatory arthritides are characterised by inflammation and damage to the joints and their surrounding structures, mediated by the immune system. It is believed that trigger factors (e.g. infection) initiate a pathological process in a susceptible individual because of genetic factors. Only a small proportion of susceptible individuals develop disease. Understanding the aetiology of rheumatic diseases requires knowledge of immunopathogenetic mechanisms, determinants of susceptibility and the nature of putative trigger factors.

Immunopathogenetic mechanisms

There are four types of immune mechanisms:

- Type I: *Allergic* reactions are mediated by IgE and provoke vasomotor and bronchospastic changes leading to asthma, urticaria or anaphylaxis
- Type II: *Cytotoxic* reactions involve cellular injury mediated by antibodies (IgG or IgM) and the activation of the complement system.
- Type III: *Immune complexes* from the circulation deposit in the tissue where they cause activation of the complement system and the generation of proinflammatory mediators.
- Type IV: *Cell mediated injury* may be mediated by T cells rather than antibodies. T cells may cause tissue injury by direct killing of cells or the elaboration of cytokines which disturb cell growth or function.

Rheumatic diseases are usually the result of type II–IV reactions, although more than one mechanism may operate concomitantly in patients.

In the initiation of the immune response, T cells recognise antigen via receptors (T-cell receptors). After activation by antigen, T cells can proliferate to serve as helper cells for B-cell antibody production or the generation of cytotoxic T cells. In addition, activated T cells can produce cytokines leading to functional changes, such as synovial cell proliferation in rheumatoid arthritis (Figure 1.1 page 15).

Susceptibility

Several factors may influence disease susceptibility (Table 1.4).

- Hormones of the neuroendocrine system can modulate immune responses, an action exploited in the use of corticosteroids as anti-inflammatory and immunosuppressive agents.

- Many rheumatic diseases show an unequal representation of the sexes, with women displaying a generally higher prevalence of inflammatory disease as well as a more serious outcome (Pisetsky 1994).
- Environmental factors may affect levels of immune cell function and together with inherited factors promote disease pathogenesis.
- Emotional and physical stress can perturb neuroendocrine function resulting in changes in immune cell function. Rheumatic diseases have long been considered to have a psychosomatic component, indicative of the belief that psychological factors influence disease onset or course (Levine et al. 1987).
- Diet may have a role in influencing disease susceptibility; in the extreme, malnutrition and serious vitamin or mineral deficiency can impair immune function. The strong influence of environmental factors on disease susceptibility can be observed by comparing disease prevalence in populations that have migrated (Solomon et al. 1975).
- Socioeconomic group and educational level also influence the susceptibility or severity of rheumatic disease, although both are likely markers for other health-related factors which include diet, occupation, lifestyle, exposure to infection, use of tobacco and alcohol and access to medical care.

Table 1.4 Factors influencing disease susceptibility

Genetic	Environment
MHC	Stress
T-cell receptor	Diet
Immunoglobulins	Drugs
Complement system components	Infection
Cytokines	
Stress responses	
Gender	

Synovitis

The synovium is the soft connective tissue lining the enclosed spaces of synovial joints, tendon sheaths and bursae. These spaces all contain a small amount of fluid rich in hyaluronic acid (synovial fluid). The functions of the synovium are:

- maintenance of an intact non-adherent tissue surface

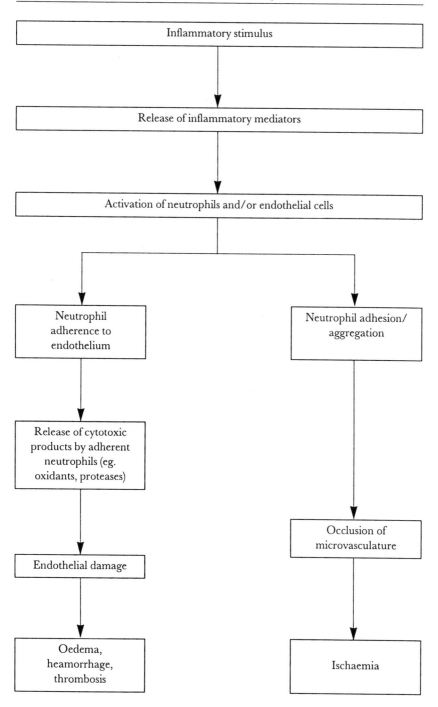

Figure 1.1 The inflammatory cascade.

- control of volume and composition of synovial fluid
- lubrication of cartilage and nutrition of chondrocytes within joints.

Inflammatory arthritides are characterised by synovitis, that is inflammation of the synovium. Acute inflammation begins when an extravascular inflammatory stimulus provokes capillary dilatation, the accumulation of plasma and fluid, and recruits circulating effector cells to the site (Figure 1.1).

Evidence is emerging that the ultimate outcome of the inflammatory response with resulting injury can be ascribed to a complex network involving products of both neutrophils and macrophages (Varani et al. 1994).

Inflamed synovium appears dramatically increased in size because of oedema, multiple redundant folds and villae. It takes on a red hue because of a dramatic increase in blood vessels. If the condition becomes chronic, synovial lining hyperplasia becomes prominent. The sublining of the synovium also undergoes dramatic alterations in the degree and content of the cellular infiltrate. The most prominent change is an exuberant infiltration with mononuclear cells, including T cells, B cells, macrophages and plasma cells. Multinucleate giant cells can be seen in granuloma-like lesions in the synovium.

1.3 Inflammatory conditions

Rheumatoid arthritis

Rheumatoid arthritis is the commonest form of chronic inflammatory joint disease. It is estimated to occur in 1–2% of the population worldwide and is a common cause of disability. It is potentially reversible if correct management is begun early (Wilske 1996). Rheumatoid arthritis is two to three times more common in women than in men. Sex differences decrease with age as the prevalence of rheumatoid arthritis appears to increase with age; by the age of 69 the sex distribution is equal (Dieppe et al. 1985). The peak age of onset varies but is commonly in the fourth and fifth decades of life.

Rheumatoid arthritis is a chronic, systemic, inflammatory, autoimmune disease of unknown aetiology. It is hypothesised that viruses, bacterial infection or psychological trauma may be initiating factors. There is a slight increase in the frequency in the condition in the first degree relatives of people who have rheumatoid arthritis. Up to 70% of people with rheumatoid arthritis test positive for HLA-DR4 antigen (le Gallez 1995).

Ryan (1997) explains that

inflammation is usually a self-limiting process – the response of the body to an offending antigen. But for reasons not fully understood, in conditions such as rheumatoid arthritis the inflammatory response becomes a continual process and can lead to destruction of much of the surrounding tissue.

As Ryan (1997) goes on to describe

whereas the complexes created by the immune system are usually ingested by the reticuloendothelial system, and deactivated once their mission is completed, in rheumatoid arthritis this does not happen. Instead, the joint lining or synovial lining proliferates, which results in pannus formation. Cartilage and tissues supporting the joints are destroyed by enzymes released as a

17

consequence of the inflammatory response. Bone is then also destroyed by the
increasing synovial membrane. As the joint space constricts, articular surfaces
are reduced and joint movement is restricted.

It has been suggested that sex hormones may also have a role in
the cause of rheumatoid arthritis (Maini and Feldman 1993).
Although their role is not entirely clear, the evidence points to the
predominance of rheumatoid arthritis in females and the increased
onset of the disease during the reproductive years and at the
menopause (le Gallez 1995). Hormones have an important influence
in women with rheumatoid arthritis. In approximately 70% of
women the manifestations of rheumatoid arthritis subside during
pregnancy and recur in the early postpartum period (Nicholas and
Panayi 1988).

Areas affected by rheumatoid arthritis

Rheumatoid arthritis is characterised by symmetrical small joint
polyarthritis involving the hands and feet, particularly the metacarpophalangeal (MCP) and the proximal interphalangeal (PIP) joints
in the hands and the metatarsophalangeal (MTP) joints in the feet.
Rheumatoid arthritis causes inflammation of the synovium which
lines both the joints and tendon sheaths of the body. As the disease
progresses other joints may also be affected, for example, the wrists,
elbows, shoulders, cervical spine, ribs, jaw (temporomandibular
joints), knees and ankles (Figure 1.2).

The course of the disease is variable, with exacerbations and
remissions over a period of time; in the majority of patients progressive joint erosions and deformity occur. Around 30% of people will
recover completely within a few years but 5% will deteriorate until
they have a significant disability (Ryan 1997).

The 1987 American Rheumatism Association Revised Criteria
for the classification of rheumatoid arthritis (Table 1.5) currently
offers the best definition of the disease in the form of a clinical
description (Arnett et al. 1988).

Rheumatoid factor

In 70–80% of patients with rheumatoid arthritis circulating rheumatoid factor (an IgM/IgG complex of two immunoglobulins) is found
in the blood (Bird et al. 1985, Ferrari et al. 1996). These patients are
classified as *seropositive*, those without a circulating rheumatoid factor
are classified as *seronegative*. However, it is important to remember

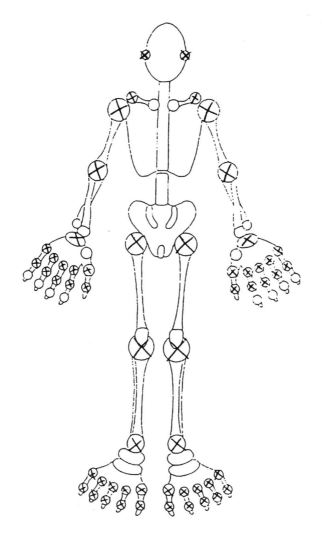

Figure 1.2 Joints affected by rheumatoid arthritis.

Table 1.5 1987 revised diagnostic criteria for the classification of rheumatoid arthritis

Morning stiffness of at least 1 hour[a]
Arthritis in at least three joint areas[b] with swelling or fluid[a]
Arthritis of hand joints (at least one area swollen in a wrist, MCP, or PIP joint)[a]
Symmetric joint swelling and involvement[a]
Subcutaneous nodules
Radiographic changes typical of rheumatoid arthritis
Positive rheumatoid factor

[a] specified criteria that must be present for at least 6 weeks.
[b] right or left proximal interphalangeal (PIP), metacarpophalangeal (MCP), wrist, elbow, knee, ankle and metatarsophalangeal (MTP) joint.

that rheumatoid factor can be detected in 5–15% of healthy subjects. Many patients who test positive for rheumatoid factor do not have rheumatoid arthritis. Other diseases commonly associated with rheumatoid factors are:

- Sjögren's syndrome
- systemic lupus erythematosus
- systemic sclerosis
- subacute bacterial endocarditis
- sarcoidosis
- chronic liver disease
- polymyositis
- acute viral infections
- parasitic infections
- tuberculosis
- syphilis (Ferrari et al. 1996).

Rheumatoid factor can be identified using the sheep cell agglutination test (SCAT), in which serum from a patient containing rheumatoid factor, heavy with immunoglobulin complexes, causes the agglutination of sheep red blood cells that have been previously coated with immunoglobulin (IgG). This test is performed at serial dilutions of the patient's serum. If a large amount of rheumatoid factor is present, flocculation of the sheep cells is likely to be observed with dilutions of the patient's serum as great as 1:256. By contrast, if only a small amount of rheumatoid factor is present flocculation will only occur with undiluted serum, or perhaps 1:8 or 1:16 (Bird et al. 1985). A positive SCAT titre of 1:80 is normally recognised as significant.

Pain and stiffness

Widespread symmetrical joint pain and swelling affecting the small peripheral joints are the commonest presenting symptoms. The immediate result of inflammation of the synovial membrane, known as *synovitis*, is a painful, stiff, hot and swollen joint. During a *'flare'* or acute attack of the disease many joints may be involved at the same time. Pain is often the first reported physical symptom, and may vary in intensity and duration from one day to the next. The patient reports early morning stiffness of variable duration and tenderness in the affected joints, which because they are swollen and painful are difficult to move, limiting the range of movement of the joints affected. The stiffness can last from a few minutes to several hours, with its duration being a guide to the level of disease activity. Muscle weakness and spasm are common in the early stages and can be followed by marked muscular atrophy.

Extra-articular manifestations

It is important to remember that the disease has an impact on the patient as a whole by affecting his or her overall physical condition, psychological wellbeing and social life. The onset of rheumatoid arthritis is usually insidious and affects the patient's body as a whole; commonly seen symptoms are general fatigue, fever, depression, weight loss and weakness. Patients may describe extreme mental and physical tiredness that is not relieved by sleep (this is caused by the inflammatory component of rheumatoid arthritis). Weight loss often occurs early in the disease, but with good disease control weight should be regained and remain stable thereafter. A normochromic or mildly hypochromic anaemia is often found in active rheumatoid arthritis. The cause seems to be a combination of poor iron intake and absorption, depression of bone marrow function, poor iron util- isation and mild haemolysis. (le Gallez 1995). Iron deficiency anaemia may also be present. Tenosynovitis and bursitis commonly accompany the disease.

Many extra-articular features of rheumatoid arthritis can occur, as listed in Table 1.6. The presence of rheumatoid nodules is often associated with a positive rheumatoid factor. They appear princi- pally on extensor surfaces or areas subjected to pressure, including the elbows, finger joints, ischial and sacral prominences, occipital scalp and Achilles tendon. They are not usually painful. Care should be taken to avoid trauma so that nodules do not become ulcerated acting as a possible source of infection. They are composed mainly of fibrinoid material (degenerative tissue cells) and granulation tissue (Judd 1997). Subcutaneous nodules may regress during treatment with disease-modifying antiarthritic drugs (DMARDs), usually as rheumatoid arthritis improves (Matteson et al. 1994). Methotrexate treatment may result in an increase in nodules, particularly over finger tendons, despite improvement in the overall disease activity (Segal et al. 1988). In general, higher concentrations of rheumatoid factor, together with the presence of nodules and radiological evidence of erosions are associated with a poorer prognosis.

Table 1.6 Extra-articular manifestations of rheumatoid arthritis

Skin	Palmar erythema
	Subcutaneous nodules
	Vasculitis
	Ulceration
Lung	Pleurisy, pleural effusions
	Pneumonitis
	Lung nodules
	Bronchiolitis obliterans
	Fibrosis
Heart	Pericarditis, pericardial effusions
	Valvular disease
	Myocarditis
Neuromuscular	Nerve entrapment
	Cervical cord compression
	Muscle wasting
	Mononeuritis multiplex
	Diffuse peripheral neuropathy
Mouth	Sicca symptoms
Eye	Episcleritis
	Scleritis, scleromalacia perforans
	Melting cornea syndrome
Haematologic	Normocytic, normochromic anaemia
	Felty's syndrome
	Amyloidosis
	Thrombocytosis
Miscellaneous	Sjögren's syndrome
	Pulmonary infections, septic arthritis
	Osteoprosis
	Tenosynovitis
	Bursitis
	Reactive lymphadenopathy
	Splenomegaly

Progression

If rheumatoid arthritis is allowed to continue uncontrolled, inflammation will eventually lead to erosion of the joint, including damage to the tendons and ligaments surrounding the joint. As the disease progresses this damage will cause the joint to become unstable, with corresponding deviation resulting in deformity (le Gallez 1995). Such deformities may include:

- radial deviation at the wrist
- ulnar deviation at the MCP joints
- palmar subluxation of proximal phalanges

- swan-neck deformity (hyperextension of PIP with flexion of DIP)
- boutonnière deformity (flexion of PIP, extension of DIP)
- hyperextension of first IP joint with flexion of first MCP (causing loss of thumb mobility and pinch)
- metatarsal prolapse
- arch collapse
- hallux valgus
- atlantoaxial subluxation (Ferrari et al. 1996).

Judd (1997) describes how instability and irritation of the joint may cause muscle contraction with resulting flexion or extension deformity or subluxation of the joint. Fibrous scar tissue and adhesions develop between the opposing joint surfaces, leading to fibrous ankylosis of the joint. The exposed, roughened ends of bone tissue may eventually proliferate bone cells into the joint cavity, resulting in calcification and bony ankylosis.

Erosions

Erosions can occur in any of the joints involved in rheumatoid arthritis; they may take many months or even years to develop. Initially, the erosions develop marginally, at the point where the synovium joins the bone, as this is the seat of inflammation (le Gallez 1995). Erosions normally occur in the MTP heads of the feet before they are seen in the MCP joints of the hands.

At the present time there is no cure for rheumatoid arthritis. The management goals include:

- control of the inflammatory process
- relief of symptoms
- prevention of joint deformity
- empowerment of the patient by assisting them to adjust to this chronic condition.

Drug treatment remains one of the major interventions in the relief of symptoms and the prevention of progress. Until the cause of rheumatoid arthritis becomes known it cannot be precisely defined. Gordon and Hastings (1994) state 'it may be one disease with more than one cause or more than one disease with a single cause'.

Juvenile idiopathic arthritis

Inflammatory joint disease is not only common in adults but in children also. Juvenile idiopathic arthritis (previously known as juvenile chronic arthritis) and known as juvenile rheumatoid arthritis in the USA, is the most common rheumatic disease of childhood and is often an important cause of disability and blindness (White 1994). In the UK the prevalence of juvenile idiopathic arthritis is approximately 10 per 100 000 of population (Symmons et al. 1996). The term is used to describe persistent arthritis affecting one or more joints which occurs in someone under 16 lasting for more than six weeks when other causes of arthritis and connective tissue disorders have been excluded (Leach 1997). It is not a single disease but rather a heterogeneous group of diseases. In patients with a diagnosis of juvenile idiopathic arthritis regular assessment by an ophthalmologist and rheumatologist is generally recommended (Ferrari et al. 1996).

Juvenile arthritis was first described by George Frederick Still, a children's specialist, in 1896. The term 'Still's disease' was used for many years with reference to childhood arthritis. It tends to be used today only to describe the rash associated with systemic onset arthritis (Leach 1997).

In very young children who cannot express their pain, the first signs may be limping, guarding of joints or even an outright refusal to move (Leach 1997).

The goals of therapy in juvenile arthritis are pain relief and preservation of joint function, so as to maintain normal growth and psychosocial development (Cassidy 1994).

Three major sub-types of juvenile idiopathic arthritis can be identified (White 1994, Leach 1997):

- *Oligoarticular onset* (55–75%): arthritis affecting fewer than five joints. The knee and ankle are the most commonly affected joints, but the small joints of the hand or the elbow can also be involved (Ansell 1977). The majority present before the age of 5 years; approximately twice as many girls are affected as boys (Leach 1997). Antinuclear antibodies are present in 40–75% of children and are associated with chronic anterior uveitis. Routine eye examination is essential (White 1994). These children are usually seronegative for rheumatoid factor (Ferrari et al. 1996). A subset of children, usually male, are HLA-B27 positive and often develop spondylitis (Leach 1997).

- *Polyarticular onset* (15–25%): arthritis affecting more than five joints. Onset is usually gradual, affecting knees, ankles, wrists and elbows. The smaller joints of the hands and feet may be affected. Most cases are seronegative; those cases that are seropositive are similar to adult onset rheumatoid arthritis and may be titled juvenile-onset adult rheumatoid arthritis (Leach 1997). This type is often positive for antinuclear antibodies.
- *Systemic onset* (Still's disease) (10–20%): presentation is with systemic features which may precede the arthritis. These may include
  - remitting fever (more than 39°C)
  - adenopathy
  - hepatosplenomegaly
  - pericarditis
  - leucocytosis
  - anaemia (Leach 1997).

There may be a rash which coincides with the peaks of fever. The arthritis usually involves multiple joints. Negative rheumatoid factor and antinuclear antibodies are typical (Ferrari et al. 1996).

The importance of juvenile idiopathic arthritis lies not in its frequency, but in the potential severity of its effects on children, and the misconceptions which surround its treatment (Southwood 1993). Southwood states that despite their limitations, children with juvenile idiopathic arthritis should be able to continue their education in the mainstream schooling system, although approximately one-third of children will still have uncontrolled arthritis or physical disabilities into adulthood.

Polymyalgia rheumatica

Polymyalgia rheumatica is a syndrome of older patients characterised by pain and stiffness in the neck, shoulders, and pelvic girdle persisting for at least 1 month (Healey 1993). It is rare before the age of 50 and becomes more common with increasing age; the cause is unknown. Morning stiffness is very prominent. There are often systemic symptoms such as anorexia, malaise, depression, fever and weight loss. Occasionally there may be synovitis of the large joints, and 10–20% of patients go on to develop temporal (giant cell) arteritis (Bird et al. 1985, Ferrari et al. 1996). Presentations of temporal arteritis can include scalp pain, pain on chewing, loss of vision in one eye or even stroke (Edwards 1991).

Diagnosis

There is no diagnostic test for polymyalgia rheumatica; the diagnosis is based on the clinical presentation. On physical examination there is little to be found other than tenderness and limited motion in the shoulders. Muscle strength is normal. Radiography is unrevealing. The erythrocyte sedimentation rate (ESR) may be very elevated and is an aid to the diagnosis. Other acute phase reactants such as C-reactive protein (CRP) and fibrinogen are also increased. Rheumatoid factor and antinuclear antibodies are not present. (Healey 1993).

The pain of polymyalgia rheumatica responds dramatically to steroids, and patients should expect to be on therapy for at least a year (Ferrari et al. 1996). The disease is usually self-limiting with a mean duration of 2 years, during this time patients may need to be on a maintenance dose of prednisolone. In those patients who develop symptoms of temporal arteritis the dose of prednisolone would be increased (Bird et al. 1985).

The clinical picture of polymyalgia rheumatica may drift towards that of rheumatoid arthritis. Here the synovitis is usually more prominent, the arthritis eventually erosive, and the response to low-dose steroids used for polymyalgia rheumatica usually insufficient (Ferrari et al. 1996).

Spondyloarthropathies

The seronegative spondyloarthropathies are characterised by:

- absence of rheumatoid factor
- a high frequency of HLA-B27 antigen positivity
- iritis
- spine and sacroiliac disease
- a variable extent of peripheral arthritis.

Conditions included in this classification are:

- ankylosing spondylitis
- psoriatic arthritis
- reactive arthritis (including Reiter's syndrome)
- bowel associated arthritis (Ferrari et al. 1996).

Ankylosing spondylitis

Ankylosing spondylitis is a chronic disorder characterised by inflammation and ensuing ankylosis of the sacroiliac joints and spinal articulations (Judd 1997). Spondylitis implies inflammation of the spine and is usually used to mean a diffuse inflammation of ligamentous insertions. This disease is more frequently seen in men than women, although an increasing number of women who do develop the disease are now recognised (Bird et al. 1985, Judd 1997).

Symptoms

Ankylosing spondylitis is characterised by stiffness in the back. Common sites are the thoracolumbar junction and low cervical region, particularly in the early morning or after a period of inactivity. The onset is usually insidious. Stiffness is initially due to inflammation, which can lead to fibrous and eventually bony ankylosis. Spondylitis is associated with sacroiliitis in nearly all cases. Patients generally find their pain improves with exercise and is worst when at rest.

An enthesopathy is responsible for many of the features of ankylosing spondylitis. It involves inflammation, fibrosis and ossification (reactive bone formation) at the enthesis (site of insertion of ligaments, tendons, and joint capsules to the bone) (Ferrari et al. 1996).

In the early stages of ankylosing spondylitis attention may be diverted from the back by complaints of aching or sharp pains in the heels, pelvis, buttocks, hips and shoulders. The back may remain silent until years after disease onset. A peripheral arthritis may occur and the arthritis may precede or follow spine disease by years.

Assessment

Examination of the spine may reveal restriction of movement. Objective assessments and spinal measurements may be undertaken to confirm and monitor this by performing a Schober's test (this assessment has been shown to correlate well with radiological movement of the lumbar spine), occiput-to-wall test, lateral flexion measurements and chest expansion measurements (Bird et al. 1985, Ferrari et al. 1996).

Iritis occurs in 20–40% of cases and has little correlation with spine disease. *Uveitis* (inflammation of the iris, ciliary body and choroid of the eye) responds well to local steroid therapy. Prompt recognition and treatment is important, and an ophthalmological opinion is therefore worthwhile (Bird et al. 1985, Ferrari et al. 1996, Judd 1997).

Other complications that may occur for patients with ankylosing spondylitis include:

- lung fibrosis
- aortitis with aortic valve regurgitation
- psoriasis
- inflammatory bowel disease.

Management

Treatment for ankylosing spondylitis consists of anti-inflammatory medication for pain relief and exercises to maintain mobility. Management has been revolutionised by the introduction of intensive exercise programmes, with close involvement from a physiotherapist, the importance of which cannot be overemphasised.

Some ankylosing spondylitis patients may require disease-modifying treatments such as sulphasalazine or methotrexate as used in rheumatoid arthritis.

Reiter's syndrome

Reiter's syndrome is a type of reactive arthritis in which certain classic extra-articular features are present. These are typically not seen in the other seronegative spondyloarthropathies. There are two variants of Reiter's syndrome. One is venereally acquired, the initial event being a urethritis which is caused by *Chlamydia*. The other is acquired from food poisoning and starts with diarrhoea, the episode following infection with *Shigella flexneri*, *Salmonella* species, *Yersinia* species or *Campylobacter* species (Bird et al. 1985, Ferrari et al. 1996). Commonly the infectious process subsides before the onset of the arthritis. Approximately 50% of patients with Reiter's syndrome will be positive for HLA-B27 antigen (Bird et al. 1985).

Symptoms

The classic triad of Reiter's syndrome refers to the presence of arthritis, urethritis and conjunctivitis, and is observed in 33% of patients (Cush and Lipsky 1993) although the majority of cases do not have all three features (Ferrari et al. 1996). The diagnosis of these patients may be identified on the basis of an acute, lower extremity oligoarthritis accompanied by one or more of the following extra-articular features: diarrhoea, urethritis, cervicitis, ocular inflammation, low back pain, enthesitis, keratoderma blennorrhagica or other mucocutaneous lesions (Cush and Lipsky 1993).

The arthropathy of Reiter's syndrome is typically an acute, asymmetric and ascending inflammatory oligoarthritis. At onset involvement of the first metatarsophalangeal, ankles, knees and toes is most common (Cush and Lipsky 1993). This is a disease of young people, males being more commonly affected than females. Involvement of the digits is sometimes accompanied by the presence of dactylitis; inflammatory swelling of a whole digit, resulting in the so-called 'sausage digit'.

Management

The aims in the management of Reiter's syndrome are:

- maintaining function
- achieving optimum joint protection
- pain relief
- suppression of inflammation
- when appropriate, eradicating infection.

For the majority of patients the initial episode of arthritis is of between 2–3 months duration, but may last up to a year. Some 20–50% of patients demonstrate a chronic course of peripheral arthritis, with the potential for progressive spondylitic changes (Cush and Lipsky 1993).

Psoriatic arthritis

Psoriatic arthritis is an inflammatory erosive arthritis associated with psoriasis, a negative rheumatoid factor and the absence of rheumatoid nodules. Dactylitis, iritis, unilateral oedema and enthesopathy (particularly around the heel) may occur. The skin manifestations may precede or follow the arthritis by many years. When arthritis antedates the skin lesions the definitive diagnosis cannot be made, and only becomes apparent with time. A family history of psoriasis should be sought. Familial aggregation suggests there is a genetic susceptibility. There is poor correlation between the severity of skin lesions and the arthritis. The sex ratio in psoriatic arthritis is close to unity.

Psoriasis is a papulosquamous, coarse scaling lesion. It may be localised (scalp, chest, periumbilicus, perianal, and extensor limb surfaces), may have accompanying pustular lesions, diffuse erythroderma and generalised exfoliative dermatitis (Ferrari et al. 1996).

Five clinical patterns of psoriatic arthritis have been recognised:

- Group 1: Predominant involvement of the *distal interphalangeal joints* (DIP). Almost always associated with psoriatic nail changes (nail pitting, onycholysis, subungual hyperkeratosis and transverse ridges – the presence of 20 pits in total suggests psoriatic arthritis, more than 60 being diagnostic).
- Group 2: *Arthritis mutilans.* This is rare. Dissolution of the bones produces shortening of the digits with redundant folds of skin, the so called *main-en-lorgnette* deformity (opera glass hands).
- Group 3: *Symmetric polyarthritis.* This is similar to rheumatoid arthritis, but with a higher frequency of DIP involvement, association with psoriasis, persistent seronegativity, associated sacroiliitis, and distinctive radiographic changes.
- Group 4: *Oligoarthritis.* This affects large joints such as knee or hip, together with one or two DIP, PIP, MCP and MTP joints, and a dactylitic or 'sausage' digit or toe.
- Group 5: *Axial involvement.* Both sacroiliitis and spondylitis can be associated with psoriatic arthritis. Spine symptoms are seldom the presenting complaint. (Bennett 1993, Helliwell and Wright 1994).

Patients with psoriatic arthritis have to bear the burden of two chronic and currently incurable diseases. They also have a dual disability in terms of employment since certain industries have self-imposed limitations on patients with any form of skin disease (Helliwell and Wright 1994). These patients require a multidisciplinary approach to give support in the emotional adjustment to the presence of arthritis and skin rash.

Methotrexate can be useful in the treatment of psoriatic arthritis as it is particularly effective in managing the skin disease as well. The use of systemic corticosteroids is avoided where possible as tapering can cause an exacerbation of the skin disease.

Inflammatory arthritis associated with infectious agents

Septic arthritis

Definition

Septic arthritis is defined as joint inflammation caused by the presence of live intra-articular micro-organisms and must be distinguished from reactive arthritis in which synovitis is triggered by a primary infection at a site distant from the joint (Hughes 1996). Hughes states that septic arthritis arises as a result of infection with bacteria, viruses, fungi, and more rarely, other more obscure micro-organisms such as protozoa.

Septic arthritis is uncommon but early diagnosis is vital to ensure that effective antimicrobial treatment may commence as delay may cause joint destruction.

Presentation

Characteristically septic arthritis has a monoarticular presentation.

- *Typical onset* is acute, with an infected joint that is warm, painful and effused. Erythema (superficial redness of the skin) may be present. The affected joint has a restricted range of movement. The patient may have a fever with chills from haematogenous bacterial entry into the joint.
- *Atypical onset* also occurs, where infection may not be obvious in joints previously damaged by prior disease that are chronically painful and swollen. Patients undergoing treatment with immunosuppressive or corticosteroid therapy are more vulnerable and may show less evidence of inflammation than other patients (Schmid 1993). Prosthetic joints are more susceptible to infection. In these joints pain that is dull, is present at night, and is described as deep and gnawing could indicate infection (Ross 1990). The appearance of sinuses or fistula and tissue necrosis surrounding prosthetic joints also suggest joint infection (Hughes 1996).

Atypical onset may be seen in children, for example, when sepsis of the hip is present it will be held immobile in flexion and abduction with little pain or swelling apparent.

Other conditions can mimic septic arthritis and should be excluded:

- crystal arthritis (gout, pseudogout)
- acute inflammatory arthritis or palindromic arthritis
- post-traumatic arthritis
- extra-articular inflammation (e.g. olecranon bursitis)
- haemarthrosis (an effusion of blood into a joint)
- rheumatic fever
- oligoarticular syndromes associated with the spondylo-arthropathies or juvenile rheumatoid arthritis.

Routes of infection

Hughes (1996) describes the five main routes by which infection of the joint in septic arthritis can occur:

- haematogenous spread, e.g. following septicaemia from wound infection, abcesses, mouth sepsis following dental procedures, recent respiratory or urogenital infection
- direct trauma, e.g. penetrating trauma with a sharp object or during a traumatic injury
- diagnostic and therapeutic procedures to a joint, e.g. joint aspiration, injection or surgical procedure such as joint replacement
- osteomyelitis
- inflamed extra-articular structures, e.g. inflamed bursae or tendon sheaths.

Micro-organisms responsible for arthritis

Almost any micro-organism can cause infectious arthritis and the aetiology will vary according to the age of the patient and other concomitant diseases present, the route of spread of infection and the distribution of joints affected. The main micro-organisms causing bacterial septic arthritis are:

- *Gram-positive cocci:* Staphylococcus aureus (the most common cause in all ages and clinical situations), Streptococcus pyogenes, Streptococcus pneumoniae, viridans-group streptococci
- *Gram-negative cocci:* Haemophilus influenzae, Neisseria gonorrhea and N. meningitidis
- *Gram-negative bacilli:* Escherichia coli, Salmonella species, Pseudomonas, coliform bacteria, Bacteroides fragilis, Brucella species, fusiform bacteria

- *Acid-fast bacilli:* Mycobacterium tuberculosis, atypical mycobacteria
- *Spirochaetes:* Leptospira icterohaemorrhagica (Hughes 1996, Schmid 1993).

Investigation and diagnosis

The history obtained should include evidence of prior or current infection elsewhere in the body; exposure to recent antibiotic treatment could mask ongoing joint infection.

Where sepsis is suspected in a joint, aspiration carried out under aseptic technique is essential so that fluid analysis can be undertaken and the diagnosis confirmed. The presence of crystals should be excluded. A high neutrophil and total white cell count in the synovial fluid raises the probability of infection. Blood cultures should be taken. Swabs should be taken, if appropriate after examination, from the ears and throat especially of children. If gonococcal infection is a possibility in adults, genital, throat and anal swabs are required.

Treatment

Patients with a definitive diagnosis of septic arthritis should be admitted to hospital for intravenous antibiotics, even before an exact identification of the infecting micro-organism is made. When culture and sensitivity results are available treatment can be changed. The duration of intravenous antibiotics will vary and long term oral antibiotics may be needed particularly for patients with prosthetic joints.

Therapy with a non-steroidal anti-inflammatory drug (NSAID) may not significantly affect septic arthritis. Corticosteroid injection is not recommended since it may significantly improve the symptoms of septic arthritis only to have joint destruction continue, and symptoms recur (Ferrari et al. 1996).

Joint aspiration and surgical joint washout is sometimes performed. Surgical removal of a prosthetic joint and all associated foreign material may be necessary if a joint replacement is confirmed as being infected. It is vital that, as soon as the patient's pain and infection are improved, mobilisation and the involvement of the physiotherapist are commenced to begin mobilising the joint and to prevent joint contractures.

Reactive arthritis

The term reactive arthritis refers to the occurrence of an acute, non-suppurative, sterile, seronegative inflammatory arthropathy that is thought to occur after exposure to an infectious agent. The infectious agent is thought to initiate an immunological response in the body, initiating a train of incompletely understood events which result in the development of synovitis at a distant site, without viable micro-organisms travelling to the joint, i.e. the infection is not active within the joints (Keat 1995, Ferrari et al. 1996). There is an association with the antigen HLA-B27 in patients with reactive arthritis. It is the commonest form of inflammatory arthritis in young men (Keat 1995).

Reiter's syndrome, already discussed, is a common type of reactive arthritis in which certain classic extra-articular features are seen. Reactive arthritis is diagnosed in the absence of the classic findings of Reiter's syndrome, the absence of psoriasis and a clear history of antecedent infection (Ferrari et al. 1996).

The onset of reactive arthritis may be insidious or acute, with associated fatigue, fever or weight loss. In a substantial number of cases, an identifiable infectious event 1–4 weeks before precedes the onset of an asymmetric oligoarthritis involving the large joints. Fifty per cent of patients present with synovitis and effusion in one or both knees (Keat 1995). Other joints less commonly affected at onset are the MTP joints, ankle joints or symptoms resulting from extensor tendinitis or enthesopathy. The infectious process subsides before the onset of the arthritis. In some patients, an identifiable infectious trigger is not apparent. Extra-articular features may include inflammatory symptoms affecting the eye, mucosal surfaces and entheses. Although reactive arthritis is frequently self-limiting it does have the potential for chronicity and articular damage (Cush and Lipsky 1993).

Triggering factors

Commonly associated and well documented with reactive arthritis are:

* gastrointestinal infections (*salmonella, shigella, yersinia, campylobacter*)
* genital tract infections (*chlamydia*).

Other infections less commonly reported are:

* bacterial: *streptococcal* (group A,G), *Clostridium difficile, Propionibacterium acne, Staphylococcus aureus* (toxic shock arthritis)
* spirochetal: *Borrelia burgdorferi* (lyme disease)

- viral: *human immunodeficiency virus (HIV)*, parvovirus
- mycobacterial: *Mycoplasma pneumoniae*
- parasitic: *Cryptosporidium* (Cush and Lipsky 1993, Keat 1995).

Information obtained during the history taking which may assist the clinician in reaching a diagnosis of reactive arthritis may be:

- a recent viral or gastrointestinal infection
- recent overseas travel (this may be associated with gastrointestinal infection)
- a new sexual partner within 3 months of onset of the arthritis (associated with genital tract infection).

Management

- Some patients whose disease is minor and short-lived may require no more than an accurate diagnosis and observation. However, the majority of patients will require treatment with a NSAID. Treatment of the original infection, where possible, with antibiotics is believed by some to be important (Ferrari et al. 1996) but is of unproven efficacy (Hughes 1996).
- Local steroid injections are useful if only one or two joints are affected and joint infection has been excluded. Steroid injection may also relieve painful enthesopathies.
- For associated urethritis or cervicitis, antibiotic therapy with tetracycline may be given, treatment is advisable for both patient and sexual partner; however, this may not influence either the duration of the arthritis or the likelihood of recurrence (Keat 1995).
- Associated bacterial diarrhoea is usually managed without antibiotics.
- Those patients with progressive disabling arthritis may require treatment with a DMARD such as methotrexate or azathioprine.

1.4
Non-inflammatory conditions

Osteoarthritis

Osteoarthritis is the commonest form of arthritis and accounts for a major amount of disability in the community (Wood 1971). It is primarily a disease of articular cartilage and subchondral bone. Focal loss of articular cartilage in part of a synovial joint is accompanied by a hypertrophic reaction in the subchondral bone and margin of the joint. There is a variable, patchy synovitis, and fibrotic thickening of the joint capsule (Figure 1.3). Radiographic changes include joint space narrowing, subchondral sclerosis and cyst formation, and marginal osteophytosis. It is an extremely common condition, which is age-related, the peak age of onset being between 50 and 60 years. Common sites which are affected include the knees, hips, distal inter-phalangeal and thumb base joints of the hands and facet joints of the spine. In all joint sites except for the hips it is commoner in women than men. There are marked racial differences in its prevalence and distribution. Clinical manifestations are use-related joint pain, stiffness of joints after a period of inactivity and loss of range of joint movement. Although age-related it is not simply an inevitable consequence of ageing but a dynamic reaction pattern of a joint responding to insult or injury. It can occur without any obvious predisposition, or it can result from a previous injury or disease of a joint (secondary osteoarthritis), hence there is great heterogeneity in the spectrum of disease covered by this term (Table 1.7). There is a lack of correlation between radiographic, pathologic and clinical manifestations and therefore attempts at strict definition have failed. The exact aetiology and pathogenesis are unknown, but are thought to involve a complex interaction of intrinsic abnormalities in connective tissue integrity and extrinsic physical insults to joints. Osteoarthritis is currently viewed as a heterogeneous disease process rather than a disease entity.

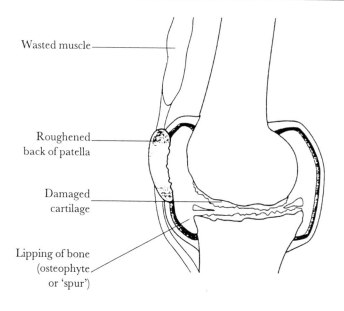

Wasted muscle

Roughened
back of patella

Damaged
cartilage

Lipping of bone
(osteophyte
or 'spur')

Figure 1.3 An osteoarthritic knee joint.

Table 1.7 Classification of osteoarthritis

Classification by the joints involved
Monoarticular, oligoarticular or polyarticular (generalized)
Chief joint site and localization within the joint
Hip (superior pole, medial pole, concentric)
Knee (medial, lateral, patellofemoral compartments)
Hand (IP joints and/or thumb base)
Spine (facet joints or intervertebral disc disease)
Others

Classification into primary and secondary[a] forms of OA
Causes of secondary OA
1. Metabolic, e.g. ochronosis, acromegaly, haemachromatosis, calcium crystal deposition
2. Anatomic, e.g. slipped femoral epiphysis, epiphyseal dysplasias, Perthe's disease, congenital dislocation of the hip, leg length inequality, hypermobility syndromes
3. Traumatic, e.g. major joint trauma, fracture through a joint, joint surgery (eg. meniscectomy), chronic injury (occupational arthropathies)
4. Inflammatory, e.g. any inflammatory arthropathy, septic arthritis

Classification by the presence of specific features
Inflammatory OA
Erosive OA
Atrophic or destructive OA
OA with chondrocalcinosis
Others

---

[a]Primary OA is idiopathic; in secondary OA a likely cause can be identified.

Fibromyalgia syndrome

Fibromyalgia is a common but often overlooked condition. It occurs predominantly in women and is associated with marked disability and handicap.

Diagnosis

Fibromyalgia syndrome presents with a variable symptom complex of widespread musculoskeletal pain (in all four quadrants), severe fatigue and multisystem 'functional' disturbance. Diagnosis is based on typical symptoms, the presence of multiple tender trigger sites (11 out of 18) and the exclusion of any inflammatory or endocrine disease. There is no specific treatment and the prognosis is often poor. Nevertheless, some patients may be helped by an explanation of the condition, limited tricyclic treatment, an increase in aerobic exercise and various coping strategies that shift the 'control' back to the patient. Medicine has a bias towards a pathological explanation of disease and fibromyalgia has often been considered an expression of psychological disturbance. The symptoms and disability, however, are real, not fabricated or imagined and reflect 'functional' rather than 'pathological' abnormality. Figure 1.4 attempts to show a possible mechanism of induction and perpetuation of fibromyalgia syndrome. Fibromyalgia may be superimposed upon pre-existing painful conditions such as osteoarthritis or cancer, although it is usually primary in nature. There is overlap in symptoms and impaired function between fibromyalgia, anxiety and depression, and fibromyalgia patients score highly on anxiety and depression questionnaires. Evidence for triggering viral infections in the vast majority of patients is lacking. Most patients are women, often in their 40s and 50s, the condition is rare in children. Pain and fatigue are often associated with severe disability. The patients may not be able to cope with their job or household activities.

Symptoms

The pain is predominantly axial and diffuse but may affect any region and at times be felt 'all over'. Characteristically the pain is not relieved by analgesics or NSAIDs. There is often a poor sleep pattern, with patients waking unrefreshed and feeling more tired in the morning than later in the day. It is important to take a full history and examination but clinical findings are usually

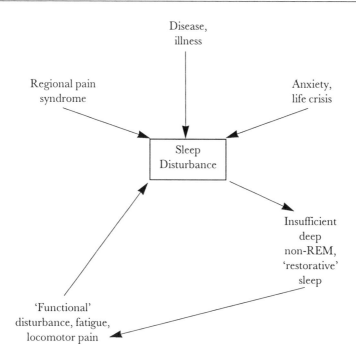

Figure 1.4 A possible mechanism of induction and perpetuation of fibromyalgia syndrome.

unremarkable with no objective weakness, synovitis or neurological abnormality. The important and sometimes the only positive examination finding is the presence of multiple hyperalgesic tender sites (Figure 1.5). These sites are tender to pressure in the normal individual but in fibromyalgia patients similar pressure elicits marked tenderness and a wince/withdrawal response. Tender sites should be found axially, in upper and lower limbs and on both sides, i.e. widespread and symmetrical. In addition hyperalgesia should be absent at control sites such as the forehead, distal forearm and fibular head.

Management

Aspects of management of fibromyalgia syndrome include:

*   patient and family education about the condition
*   trial of tricyclics
*   cessation of other ineffective drugs
*   graded aerobic exercise regime
*   coping strategies, e.g. yoga.

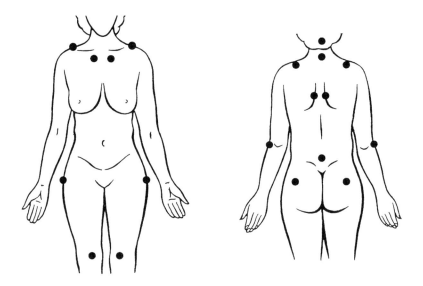

Figure 1.5 Common hyperalgesic tender sites.

The prognosis is poor, with less than 1 in 10 patients in a study in Nottingham losing their symptoms over a 5-year period. With suitable advice patients, although not 'cured', can learn to live better with their condition and more importantly avoid further unnecessary investigations and drug treatments (Doherty 1993).

1.5 Connective tissue disease

The connective tissue diseases are a group of multisystem diseases frequently characterised by pathologic changes in blood vessels and connective tissues. These diseases often have overlapping clinical features and share immunological abnormalities, including:

* general systemic features (malaise, weight loss, fever)
* musculoskeletal involvement varying from inflammatory polyarthritis to generalised arthralgia and myalgia
* immune aberration leading to immune-mediated inflammation as an underlying pathogenic mechanism (Kimberly and Urowitz 1994).

Systemic lupus erythematosus

Systemic lupus erythematosus is an inflammatory, multisystem disease of unknown aetiology with diverse clinical and laboratory manifestations and a variable course and prognosis. Immunological aberrations give rise to excessive production of autoantibodies, some of which cause cytotoxic damage, while others participate in immune complex formation resulting in immune inflammation.

Clinical manifestations may be constitutional or result from inflammation in various organ systems including skin and mucous membranes, joints, kidney, brain, serous membranes, lung, heart and occasionally gastrointestinal tract. Organ systems may be involved individually or in any combination. Involvement of vital organs (particularly kidneys and central nervous system) accounts for significant morbidity and mortality. Morbidity and mortality result from tissue damage due to the disease process or its therapy. Systemic lupus erythematosus is recognised worldwide, but its prevalence varies in different geographic areas. It is more prevalent in women, particularly in their reproductive years. In the US it has been noted that the disease is three times more common among blacks than whites.

Symptoms

Clinical features of systemic lupus erythematosus include:

- *general constitutional complaints:* (weight loss, fever, malaise, over-whelming fatigue).
- *skin manifestations* (lupus-specific or lupus-non-specific):
  acute lupus-specific lesions: malar rash, generalised erythema, bullous lupus erythematosus
  subacute lupus-specific lesions:
  - chronic lupus changes localised discoid, generalised discoid, lupus profundus
- *photosensitivity* (over 50% of patients)
- *alopecia* (patchy or diffuse)
- *mucous membrane lesions* (ulcers of the mouth or vagina or nasal septal erosions).
- *musculoskeletal features* (arthralgias and/or arthritis): often the presenting manifestation. The acute arthritis typically involves the small joints of the hands, wrists and knees. Most cases are symmetrical. Nodules are found in 10% of cases. Unlike rheumatoid arthritis, the arthritis of systemic lupus erythematosus is typically not erosive or destructive of bone. However, clinical deforming arthritis does occur and may take a number of different forms; there may be mild synovial thickening about PIP joints or over tendon sheaths, ulnar deviation of the fingers and subluxations and contractures. Patients may complain of muscle pain and weakness. This may be due to arthritis, be drug-induced (corticosteroids, antimalarials) or due to true muscle inflammation (polymyositis).
- *Renal disease:* urinalysis and serum creatinine assessments must be made regularly. Renal biopsy may be needed to assess the lupus nephritis accurately.
- *Neuropsychiatric manifestations:* patients often present with a mixture of neurological and psychiatric manifestations.
- *Neurological manifestations:* seizures, headache, transverse myelitis, cranial or peripheral neuropathy.
- *Psychiatric manifestations:* psychosis, psychoneurosis and neurocognitive dysfunction.
- *Serositis:* pleurisy, pericarditis, peritonitis.

- *Pulmonary involvement:* lupus pleuritis, lupus pneumonitis, pulmonary haemorrhage, pulmonary embolism, pulmonary hypertension.
- *Cardiac involvement:* pericarditis, myocarditis, endocarditis, coronary artery disease.
- *Gastrointestinal involvement:* oesophageal disease, mesenteric vasculitis, inflammatory bowel disease, pancreatitis, liver disease.
- *Haematological abnormalities:* anaemia, leucopenia or lymphopenia and thrombocytopenia. The most significant anaemia is the autoimmune haemolytic anaemia due to autoantibodies directed against red blood cell antigens. The lupus anticoagulant is the commonest haemostatic abnormality. The serology of lupus shows evidence for complement consumption by immune complexes. Antibodies seen in systemic lupus erythematosus include antinuclear antibodies, anti-smooth muscle, anti-Ro, anti-La and antibodies to double-stranded DNA.

There is a greater incidence of spontaneous abortion, prematurity and interuterine death, although systemic lupus erythematosus does not interfere with conception. Survival rates have improved over the last four decades from less than 50% at 5 years in 1955 to over 90% survival at 5 years in 1990. Reasons for this improvement include earlier diagnosis, better therapeutic modalities, improved antibiotics and antihypertensive drugs and the availability of renal dialysis and transplantation (Gladman and Urowitz 1994).

Scleroderma (systemic sclerosis)

Scleroderma is a generalised disorder of connective tissue affecting skin and internal organs. It is characterised by fibrotic arteriosclerosis of peripheral and visceral vasculature. Variable degrees of extracellular matrix accumulation occur (mainly collagen), both in skin and viscera. It is associated with specific autoantibodies, most notably anticentromere and Scl-70.

Systemic sclerosis is a remarkably heterogeneous disorder, with diverse initial presentations and variable disease course. Periodic waxing and waning of symptoms is unusual (unlike rheumatoid arthritis or systemic lupus erythematosus).

Clinical features

- Raynaud's phenomenon
- tightening and thickening of skin (scleroderma)
- involvement of internal organs, including gastrointestinal tract,

lungs, heart and kidneys, accounts for increased morbidity and mortality
• risk of internal organ involvement strongly linked to extent and progression of skin thickening.

The first convincing description of scleroderma was of a 17-year-old woman in Naples in 1753 (Rodnan and Benedek 1962). The relationship of scleroderma to Raynaud's phenomenon was first described by Maurice Raynaud himself in 1865. In 1945 Goetz proposed the term *progressive systemic sclerosis*, based on his detailed review of the visceral lesions (Goetz 1945). The aetiology and pathogenesis remain unknown and no effective therapies for the basic disorder have been developed. Breakthroughs in treatment of specific clinical features have derived from agents developed for other purposes and include angiotensin-converting enzyme (ACE) inhibitors for the hypertension associated with renal involvement and histamine-2 (H_2) receptor antagonists for chronic acid reflux.

Epidemiology

Studies based on hospital records and death registries suggest occurrence in between 4 and 12 individuals per million population per year. It is likely that many cases of systemic sclerosis are unrecognised, particularly in limited disease. Onset is highest in the fourth and fifth decade of life and is 3–4 times more common in women than in men (Medsger and Masi 1971). Disease is not linked to race, season, geography, occupation or socioeconomic status. Environmental aetiologies are possible and implicated factors include silica dust, silicone surgical implants and epoxy resins. Familial occurrence is quite rare and convincing genetic associations are lacking.

Vascular abnormalities

• *Raynaud's phenomenon*. This is defined as episodic colour changes (pallor, cyanosis, erythema) occurring in response to environmental cold and/or emotional stress. Although most typically noted in the fingers, the circulation of the toes, ears, nose and tongue is also frequently affected. Subjects complain of symptoms of numbness and pain associated with the phases of pallor and cyanosis and of tingling and burning during the hyperaemic recovery phase. The impact on hand function in cold environments can be substantial. Raynaud's phenomenon is the initial complaint in around three-quarters of patients with systemic sclerosis and its potential importance in systemic sclerosis cannot be understated. Taken alone it has considerable clinical impact; however, abnormalities similar to those of the peripheral circulation are widely distributed in the visceral vasculature as well and have major effects on morbidity and mortality. In systemic sclerosis structural narrowing of the digital arteries causes severe (>75%) attenuation of the arterial lumen. The principal lesion is one of intimal hyperplasia consisting of collagen. Lesser degrees of fibrosis are noted in the adventitia but the media (smooth muscle) is little affected. Normal peripheral vasoconstriction in response to cold superimposed on the narrowed vessel would cause occlusion of the lumen. Similarly, treatment of Raynaud's phenomenon with smooth muscle relaxants is less likely to work in the presence of a fixed obstructive lesion. The hallmark of severity of Raynaud's phenomenon in systemic sclerosis is the frequency of digital ischaemic injury. Around one-third of patients experience at least one digital ulceration per year and patients are at risk of catastrophic peripheral digital gangrene. Modern clinical studies suggest that the internal organs sustain Raynaud-like intermittent ischaemia during cold exposure (heart, lungs).

- *Microvascular abnormalities.* There are characteristic architectural abnormalities of the microvasculature in systemic sclerosis which are easily appreciated by widefield microscopy of the nailfold capillary bed (Maricq 1981). These changes include enlargement and tortuosity of individual capillary loops interspersed with areas of capillary loop dropout. At later stages of clinical disease, punctate telangiectasias develop with typical locations including fingers, face, lips and oral mucosa.

Skin involvement

The early tissue lesion features ingress of immigrant inflammatory cell populations. The net effect of this array of cells and signals is accumulation of extracellular matrix including collagen glycosaminoglycan, fibronectin, adherence molecules and tissue water. The patient and clinician recognise the result as the tightened and thickened skin (scleroderma) which is the hallmark of disease.

- *Oedematous change.* An intrinsic feature of early systemic sclerosis is the painless swelling of the fingers and hands. Symptoms include early morning stiffness and arthralgia. *Carpal tunnel syndrome* is a frequent occurrence. Pitting oedema of the fingers and dorsum of the hand is present on examination.
- *Scleroderma.* Skin thickening begins on the fingers and hands in virtually all cases. The skin initially appears shiny and taut and may be erythematous. Pruritus is common and may be intense. Digital skin creases are obscured and hair growth is reduced. The skin of the face and neck is usually involved next. Facial scleroderma causes an immobile and pinched facies. The lips become thin and pursed. The local skin thickening limits the ability to open the mouth fully, impairing effective dental hygiene. Skin thickening may stay limited to hands and face, but in some patients there is rapid spread to the upper arms, shoulders, chest, back, abdomen and legs. Prominent localised areas of hyperpigmentation and hypopigmentation may develop.
- *Skin thickening and disease classification.* The diagnosis of systemic sclerosis is clinically obvious once skin thickening has developed. Accurate and early classification is the paramount clinical issue because the relative risk of accruing new internal organ involvement closely parallels the pace, progression and extent of skin involvement (Table 1.8).
- *Skin, visceral involvement and disease outcome.* Skin involvement alone is symptomatic and by virtue of local tethering contributes to loss of motion, impaired hand function, cosmetic problems and lessened sense of well being (McCloskey et al. 1990). The importance of skin involvement stems from its linkage with visceral changes.

Table 1.8 Classification of systemic sclerosis

I	Diffuse scleroderma – skin thickening present on the trunk in addition to the face, proximal and distal extremities
II	Limited scleroderma – skin thickening restricted to sites distal to the elbow and knee, but also involving the face and neck Synonym – CREST syndrome (calcinosis, Raynaud's, oesophageal dysmotility, sclerodactyly, telangiectasias)
III	Sine scleroderma – no clinically apparent skin thickening but with characteristic internal organ changes, vascular and serologic features
IV	In overlap – criteria fulfilling systemic sclerosis occurring concomitantly with criteria fulfilling diagnoses of SLE, RA or inflammatory muscle disease
V	Undifferentiated connective tissue disease – Raynaud's phenomenon with clinical and/or laboratory features of systemic sclerosis

Systemic features

- *General manifestations.* Fever is uncommon, and its presence should prompt a search for infection. Weight loss is universal even in the absence of gastrointestinal involvement. Profound fatigue occurs frequently and is often a limiting factor in daily activities. Both the unrelenting persistence of symptoms and concern over the cosmetic impact of the disease lead to frequent reactive depression. Systemic sclerosis is uncommon; many patients have not heard of the disease prior to their diagnosis.

- *Gastrointestinal involvement.* This is the third most common feature following Raynaud's phenomenon and scleroderma. Incompetence of the lower oesophageal sphincter is suggested by symptoms of heartburn and associated bitter regurgitation. Impaired contractility of the smooth muscle of the oesophagus presents as dysphagia and odynophagia for solid foods. Complaints of a 'sticking' sensation are typical. Small intestine involvement is a major source of morbidity. Symptoms include intermittent bloating with abdominal cramps, intermittent or chronic diarrhoea and presentations of intestinal obstruction. Malabsorption can be shown by an increased quantitative faecal fat elimination. Bacterial overgrowth in areas of intestinal stasis is well documented.

- *Musculoskeletal features.* The majority of patients experience arthralgia and morning stiffness. Overt arthritis is uncommon; erosive arthropathy is demonstrable on radiograph in 20–30% of patients (Blocka et al. 1981). Inflammatory and fibrinous involvement of tendon sheaths may mimic arthritis. Muscle weakness occurs both from disuse atrophy and from a disease-related myopathy. Resorption of bone of the digital tufts occurs in longstanding disease. Subcutaneous calcinosis can occur, common locations include the fingers, preolecranon area, olecranon and prepatellar bursae. These areas become intermittently inflamed and a source of discomfort. Spontaneous extrusion through the skin is a frequent occurrence and a source of local infection.

- *Pulmonary involvement.* Pulmonary involvement is the leading cause of mortality and morbidity in later stages of systemic sclerosis. Any combination of vascular obliteration, fibrosis and inflammation may be present. Clinical presentations are insidious and include exertional dyspnoea, diminished exercise tolerance and non-productive cough. Pulmonary function testing is the mainstay of clinical diagnosis and serial assessment.

- *Myocardial involvement.* Patchy fibrosis of the myocardium is present at autopsy in as many as 81% of patients with systemic sclerosis. Myocardial involvement is a principal determinant of survival. Many patients complain of diminished exercise tolerance, palpitations and dyspnoea and therefore separating myocardial from pulmonary involvement in clinical assessment is difficult.
- *Renal involvement.* The syndrome of 'scleroderma renal crisis' is due to the sudden onset of accelerated hypertension, rapidly progressive renal insufficiency, microangiopathic haemolysis and consumptive thrombocytopenia in the presence of hyperreninaemia.
- *Pregnancy.* Menstrual irregularities and amenorrhoea occur in relation to the severity of illness. Difficulty with conception is frequent. Pregnancy is not associated with worsening of scleroderma.

Immunological features

Systemic sclerosis occurs in overlap with other connective tissue disorders including systemic lupus erythematosus, polymyositis, rheumatoid arthritis and Sjögren's syndrome. Antinuclear antibodies are present in the sera of over 90% of patients with systemic sclerosis.

Inflammatory muscle disease (polymyositis)

Definition

Inflammatory muscle disease is a member of the connective tissue disease family (autoimmune disease associations, other immunological features), characterised by chronic inflammation of striated muscle (polymyositis) and sometimes the skin (dermatomyositis). Autoantibody associations define clinical subsets of the disease.

Clinical features

Clinical features of inflammatory muscle disease include:
- painless proximal muscle weakness with or without rash
- elevation of serum muscle enzymes (creatine kinase)
- other organ systems affected (joints, lungs, heart, gastrointestinal tract)
- probable association with malignancy (in elderly people).

Epidemiology

Classification of these diseases is being refined as new insights into aetiology and pathogenesis emerge. These disorders are recognised as part of a single disease spectrum. Certain features are used to separate subsets:

- childhood versus adult onset
- polymyositis versus dermatomyositis
- presence or absence of other connective tissue diseases or malignancy.

In the future it is likely that disease subsets will be identified according to serum autoantibodies and/or other immunologic characteristics.

Incidence

The annual incidence of polymyositis/dermatomyositis ranges from 2 to 10 new cases per million persons at risk in various populations. Published rates are likely to be underestimates as not all possible sources of ascertainment are examined.

Inflammatory myopathy can occur at any age but the observed pattern of incidence includes childhood and adult peaks. The incidence sex ratio is 2.5:1 female to male. This ratio is 1:1 in childhood disease and associated malignancy but 10:1 when there is an associated connective tissue disease. Polymyositis/dermatomyositis has a 3–4:1 black/white incidence ratio.

Environmental factors

Inflammatory myopathy has no striking associations with environmental factors.

- Onset more frequent in winter and spring months (precipitation by viral and bacterial infections).
- D–penicillamine (drug induced myositis).

Genetic factors

At least in some families there seems to be a genetic predisposition. It is not uncommon to find close relatives who suffer from other autoimmune diseases (Walker et al. 1982). The reported associations of certain HLA types with clinical subsets of disease are weak.

Presentations

The presentation of inflammatory muscle disease is characterised by:

- insidious, progressive, painless proximal muscle weakness over 3–6 months
- acute onset muscle pain and weakness developing over several weeks (associated with fever and fatigue)
- proximal myalgias only
- slowly evolving weakness over 5–10 years (inclusion body myositis).

Signs and symptoms

- *Constitutional:* fatigue, fever and weight loss.
- *Skeletal muscle:* Patients complain of difficulty performing activities of daily living requiring normal muscle strength. Walking may become clumsy, with a 'waddling' gait. Bulbar weakness results in hoarseness or dysphonia, difficulty in initiating swallowing with regurgitation of liquids and episodic coughing immediately after swallowing. Physical examination is necessary to confirm weakness of individual muscles or groups of muscles. The distribution of weakness is usually symmetric, affecting all proximal muscles. Distal muscles are only weak in 10–20% of cases. Ocular and facial muscles are rarely involved. Swelling of muscle is usual. Firmness to touch and incomplete passive stretching suggest fibrous replacement of muscle and contractures respectively.
  - Skin
    Dermatomyositis: erythematous or violaceous, scaling, oedema, cuticular hypertrophy and haemorrhage, periungual erythema and telangiectasia, ulceration
    Polymyositis/dermatomyositis: panniculitis, cutaneous mucinosis, vitiligo, multifocal lipoatrophy

Other features

- *Joints:* polyarthralgias and/or polyarthritis which are rheumatoid-like in distribution. Wrists, knees and small joints of the hands are most frequently affected. Arthritis tends to occur early in the disease and is mild and transient (Schumacher et al. 1979).

- *Calcinosis* can be a late problem in polymyositis/dermatomyositis. Intracutaneous, subcutaneous and fascial sites are affected, as well as the connective tissue surrounding muscle bundles.
- *Respiratory involvement:* dyspnoea on exertion may be due to respiratory muscle (diaphragm, intercostal) weakness. It may be due to congestive heart failure or cardiac arrythmia from myocardial or conduction system involvement. Intrinsic causes of dyspnoea include interstitial alveolitis or fibrosis, aspiration pneumonia (from pharyngeal dysmotility), bacterial infection and methotrexate pulmonary toxicity (Dickey and Myers 1984). Cough is frequent. There are three common presentations of lung disease:
  - aggressive form of diffuse alveolitis (myositis often overlooked)
  - slowly progressive lung disease (disability from myopathy may mask severity of lung disease)
  - asymptomatic but with radiographic and/or physiologic manifestations of interstitial lung disease
- *Cardiac involvement* is common but seldom symptomatic until it is very advanced. The most frequent abnormality is a rhythm disturbance. Less common is congestive heart failure due to myocarditis or fibrous replacement of the myocardium.
- *Gastrointestinal tract:* pharyngeal dysphagia can occur. Involvement of the smooth muscle of the intestinal tract is uncommon unless there is overlap with systemic sclerosis. Lower oesophageal dysphagia results in the sensation of food 'sticking' in the retrosternal area during the act of swallowing. A weak lower oesophageal sphincter leads to reflux of gastric acid causing heartburn. Chronic distal oesophagitis predisposes to stricture formation. Constipation is the most common symptom of colonic hypomotility.
- *Peripheral vasculature:* Raynaud's phenomenon is a frequent accompanying complaint.
- *Association with malignancy:* the relationship between myositis and malignancy is controversial. Cancer in myositis patients is most frequently obvious rather than occult.

Investigations

- *General:* low-grade anaemia is present in polymyositis (anaemia of chronic disease). ESR may be mildly elevated.

Musculoskeletal

- *Enzymes from injured skeletal muscle:* creatine kinase, aldolase, the transaminases (ALT and AST) and lactate dehydrogenase.
- *Electromyogram* (EMG) is a sensitive but non-specific method of evaluating inflammatory myopathy. Typical findings include irritability of myofibrils on needle insertion and at rest and short duration, low amplitude, complex potentials on contraction. The EMG is a useful method for following disease activity.
- *Muscle biopsy* should be performed in all cases to confirm the diagnosis of inflammatory myopathy. The presence of chronic inflammatory cells in the perivascular and interstitial areas surrounding myofibrils is pathognomonic. More common than inflammation are degeneration and necrosis of myofibrils, phagocytosis of necrotic cells and myofibril regeneration. In long-standing myositis, fibrous connective tissue replaces necrotic myofibres and separates bundles of myofibres.

- *Lung:* reduced respiratory muscle strength is determined by measuring inspiratory pressures at the mouth. The chest radiograph in interstitial lung disease shows bilateral basilar thickening. Thin section computerized axial tomography (CT) reveals evidence of interstitial fibrosis. Ventilation–perfusion studies are abnormal and pulmonary function tests show a restrictive physiologic pattern with reduced forced vital capacity.
- *Heart:* the most common alterations are conduction defects and atrial and ventricular dysrhythmias which are due to involvement of working myocardium and/or the conducting system.
- *Intestine:* barium studies are used to demonstrate pharyngeal dysphagia, delayed gastric emptying and small bowel dilatation and hypomotility.
- *Serum autoantibodies:* in polymyositis/dermatomyositis over 80% of patients have autoantibodies to nuclear and/or cytoplasmic antigens (antinuclear antibodies, ANCA). 50% of patients have myositis-specific antibodies, which may be important in the pathogenesis of the inflammatory myopathies (association with subsets, selective response against antigens, variation of antibody titre with disease activity).

Natural history

The majority of patients have multiple exacerbations and remissions or persistent disease activity. With each episode of myositis there is the potential for absolute loss of muscle mass.

Prognosis

Assessment of prognosis is difficult because the disease is relatively rare, a classification system based on meaningful pathophysiologic and serologic data has not been developed, and objective criteria for improvement (or deterioration) are not standardised.

Survival

Since the availability of corticosteroids there has been improved survival, although there have been no double-blind placebo-controlled studies. Currently the expected survival in incident cases of polymyositis/dermatomyositis is over 90% at 5 years after initial diagnosis. Factors associated with poor survival include:

- older age
- malignancy
- delayed initiation of corticosteroid therapy
- pharyngeal dysphagia with aspiration pneumonia
- myocardial involvement
- complications of corticosteroid or immunosuppressive drugs.

Disability

Each major exacerbation results in a reduction in muscle strength, but therapy almost never returns the patient to the preceding level of total body muscle mass or strength. Fortunately a minor amount of atrophy and weakness in one or more muscle groups most often does not translate into functional impairment.

1.6 Impact of rheumatological conditions on everyday functioning: physical, social, psychological and occupational

Over 200 conditions affecting joints, bones, soft tissues and muscles are covered by the term arthritis, often referred to as 'rheumatic disease' or 'musculoskeletal disease' (Symmons and Bankhead 1994). Arthritis is the biggest cause of physical disability in the UK (Martin et al. 1988).

The two main types of arthritis in terms of diagnosis are:

- non-inflammatory, e.g. osteoarthritis
- inflammatory – e.g. rheumatoid arthritis.

Rheumatoid arthritis is characterised by progressive disability over time. Using the Stanford Health Assessment Questionnaire (HAQ) it has been clearly demonstrated that functional status deteriorates over time (Doyle 1996). Research has shown that disability occurs early in the course of the disease (Wolfe and Cathey 1991, Wolfe et al. 1991).

The impact and personal costs of rheumatological conditions on the individual and their family, in terms of pain, loss of physical movement, loss of independence, self-esteem, employment, education, disruption to relationships, reduced quality of family and social life is incalculable (Aschroft 1997).

The current aim of medical care, in the absence of a cure, is a reduction in the impact of rheumatoid arthritis. Although some accept that there is a need to consider and take into account the impact of the disease on the individual's social functioning (Long and Scott 1994), health professionals tend to work within the medical model of disability and aim to establish 'what works on whom, and why' (Ashcroft 1996). However, the impact of a chronic rheumatological condition on the quality of life for both individuals and their families should not be ignored. Carr (1996) states that quality of life measures are required to identify and assess the disabling consequences of rheumatoid arthritis and the effectiveness of medical attempts to prevent or postpone them.

In 1980 The World Health Organisation provided definitions of impairment, disability and handicap in an attempt to distinguish between the clinical and social consequences associated with a chronic disease (WHO 1980). Measurement tools to assess impairment and disability are well established in the field of rheumatology; quality of life measurement tools to assess the consequences suffered by an individual as a result of a disease or handicap are not.

Carr (1996) tells us that 'handicap is the social consequence of disease, is specific to individuals and depends not only on the severity of the disease, but also on his or her life role'. She goes on to say that 'the degree to which an individual is handicapped depends on the perception of the importance of the role that can no longer be filled'. Discrepancies between the views of society (employers, health care professionals) and individuals with regard to handicaps can be considerable.

Personal impact of arthritis

It must be remembered that rheumatoid arthritis affects the patient's body as a whole, not just the articular system, and invariably has an impact on every aspect of the patient's physical and psychosocial life (Gordon and Hastings 1994).

The impact of a rheumatological condition can be felt even before a diagnosis has been made, when due to pain and stiffness in the joints performing everyday activities of daily living, like washing, dressing and cooking are both painful and difficult. From a patient's perspective Ashcroft (1996) describes how

> an early diagnosis brings with it a never ending stream of appointments with consultants, doctors, occupational therapists, physiotherapists, blood tests, X–rays, trips to the GP and chemist etc. This, coupled with the extreme fatigue

that accompanies rheumatoid arthritis, leads to your entire life being absorbed within the medical world.

She goes on to describe how this

represents the insidious nature of rheumatoid arthritis, sucking you very quickly into an 'illness mode' – the medical model of disability, and like most things held in by suction, it is very difficult, if not impossible to get back out.

It is vital that health professionals ensure adequate information is given to every patient, either newly diagnosed or with established disease, to enable them to understand what type of arthritis they have, its course and how it may progress and how they can learn to manage their condition themselves.

Diagnosis can bring about many emotions – denial, relief or disbelief to name but a few. It might be assumed that anxiety and depression would correlate with continuing disease activity, but it appears that socioeconomic factors may be greater determinants of depression than physical factors (Hawley and Wolfe 1988, McFarlane and Brooks 1988).

Age factors

The impact of the diagnosis will affect not only the individual but family and friends also and being diagnosed with arthritis at various age groups will have different implications (Ashcroft 1997).

*   *Young children* with arthritis may become withdrawn, isolated and depressed if they are not able to join their friends in normal childhood school, playground and recreational activities. Schooling may be disrupted. Friction may develop with other siblings if they perceive more attention is given to the 'disabled' child by parents. (see also 'Impact on education', below.)
*   *Teenagers*, although nearing independence, may require assistance because of physical limitations and may need help with personal care, which is difficult to come to terms with both for parent and child. The attainment of independence, physical maturity, social and sexual identity may all be delayed. Depression and anxiety may become problems. Parents can then become overprotective.
*   *Young adults* may no longer be able to pursue their chosen career ambition. (see also 'Impact on employment, below.)
*   *Middle aged adults:* arthritis can curtail a successful career or

prompt an unwanted change of direction. A reduction of income may result. Taking time off work may be necessary and can affect relationships with workmates.

For any age group the impact on long term relationships can be the greatest. Ashcroft (1997) explains 'the spontaneity of a hug can cause excruciating pain and the reaction to being the cause of that pain is often guilt'. Tensions can easily develop within a relationship.

The fluctuating nature of arthritis can be a contributory factor to stress within the family and workplace as people find it difficult to understand the ability to do a thing one day and not the next.

Financial impact

To individuals and their families, living with arthritis can be expensive. Extra expenses incurred can include:

- additional heating and hot water
- personal assistance and care
- domestic help
- household and garden maintenance
- home adaptations
- specialist equipment – lever taps, lever door handles, electric tin openers, bottle and jar openers, aids to assist with washing and dressing, aids to assist with preparing and cooking food
- mobility – taxi or bus fares, car adaptations such as power assisted steering, automatic transmission, electric windows, central locking, hand brake adaption
- prescription and non-prescription medicines.

Impact on education

Two important principles are at stake in the education of a child with arthritis (Southwood 1993):

- the child should be made to feel as independent and normal as possible
- keeping the child in mainstream schooling is crucial.

The child with arthritis may have a decreased attention span, irritability, increased sleepiness and altered mood secondary to the disease itself or its treatment (Southwood 1993).

It should be possible for children who need to spend time in hospital or at home to continue their education. Liaison between parents, school and hospital teachers and individual tutors is important to ensure a work plan is formulated. Minimal disruption is desirable to ensure career choices are not prejudiced at a later date.

Children with arthritis may have pain and stiffness in their hands which may cause slowness and difficulty in writing. They should be allowed extra time to complete work, and consideration for the use of a word processor, electric typewriter or tape recorder may be useful.

Mobility and movement in general may be a problem and extra time should be allocated, if necessary, for carrying books from one classroom to another.

It may not be possible for children with arthritis to participate fully in physical education lessons, but close liaison with a physiotherapist who can suggest appropriate exercises is useful. Swimming is excellent, provided the pool is not too cold. Contact sports, which may cause direct injury to a joint are not usually advisable, noncontact sports are preferred.

A patient's educational background and occupation may affect management and outcome. Notwithstanding genetic and sex factors, patients with more years of education seem to develop less severe disease (Leigh and Fries 1991). Hilliquin and Menkes (1994) describe how relationships between education and outcome in rheumatoid arthritis are not well understood. They go on to explain how low formal education appears to be a marker identifying behavioural risk factors that may be associated with a poor outcome in rheumatoid arthritis. These factors include the patient's sense of self-efficacy, problem-solving capacity, sense of personal responsibility and capacity to cope with life stress. Patients with less schooling may not know where to turn for help, may seek medical care less promptly and report to physicians later in the course of the disease. Compliance with treatments could also be reduced.

Impact on employment

The onset of arthritis, particularly inflammatory arthritis, may result in a change of a chosen career path. Some people who developed their arthritis at a young age may have difficulty gaining employment, whereas some people with arthritis may have to stop work altogether. Some the pain and fatigue associated with arthritis, which may be exacerbated by stress, affects the hours of work they can manage. Gordon and Hastings (1994) claim that people whose occupations are associated with less physical stress show a better functional outcome.

Individuals should be encouraged to discuss with their employers, at an early stage, modifications or adjustments that could reasonably be made to make it easier for them to carry out their work. Practical help and support is available to employers through the government's Access to Work scheme. This scheme is administered by the Employment service through local placing, assessment and counselling teams (PACTs).

Being able to gain and retain employment is not easy at the best of times and for people with arthritis it can be more difficult. However, it is important to remember that all people, whether or not they have arthritis, are individuals and will bring their own skills, strengths and weaknesses to their work.

Role of social support in rheumatic disease

As already mentioned, coping with rheumatic disease involves facing a number of stresses and challenges. In addition to coming to terms with the meaning of the illness for one's life and the more emotive issues of disease progression and deformity, individuals must cope with pain, stiffness and activity restrictions on a daily basis. Many of these adaptive challenges require help from others. Thus, for patients with rheumatic disease, an available and satisfying network of interpersonal relations, on which they can count for both emotional support and more practical assistance during periods of pain and disability, is essential.

Rheumatic disease has an inevitable impact on the patient's family. The emotional reactions of patients to their illness spill over into feelings of helplessness and distress among family members. The fluctuating nature of many of the rheumatic conditions means family members must learn when to give and when to withhold help, as providing too much support or providing it at the wrong time may produce negative outcomes (Revenson 1990).

Impact on family relationships

Rheumatic disease can affect the family in many ways. Some patients report their arthritis brings them closer as a family, some say it makes no difference and others feel it has a negative effect on family life.

- *The spouse and the marriage.* There is conflicting evidence as to whether the divorce rate is higher in patients with rheumatic disease, whether illness precipitates divorce or whether the lower rate of remarriage is associated with disease course (Medsger and Robinson 1972). There is no dispute that rheumatic disease causes stress for the healthy spouse and on the marriage. Stressors caused by the conditions create demands for increased emotional support and tangible assistance from the healthy partner. Responsibilities may move outside traditional gender roles (Staines 1986). As well as the patient possibly feeling more anxious and depressed, the spouses of ill individuals often experience depression and anxiety, marriage communication difficulties and problems at work (Flor et al. 1987).
- *Effects of parent's disease on children.* In one study adolescents with a parent who had arthritis had poorer self-esteem than the comparison group (no parental disorder) (Hirsch et al. 1985). It has been suggested that for adolescents whose parents have arthritis, involvement of friends with their families presents more opportunities for friends to 'see the disability', and consequently evaluate the parent, and by extension, the adolescent negatively. Thus, the parent's physical disability might have a negative impact on the adolescent's ability to draw on friendships for support (Hirsch and Reischl 1985).
- *Benefits of social support.* Arthritis patients receiving more support from friends and family exhibit greater self-esteem (Fitzpatrick et al. 1988), psychological adjustment (Affleck et al. 1988) and life satisfaction (Burckhardt 1985). They cope more effectively with the illness (Manne and Zautra 1989) and show less depression (Fitzpatrick et al. 1988). Support from family members may also enhance compliance with treatment interventions (Radojevic et al. 1992).
- *Costs of receiving social support.* Receiving, using or requesting social support has its costs as well as its benefits (Revenson and Majerovitz 1990). The costs of asking for or receiving help involve threats to self-esteem, loss of autonomy and decreased psychological well-being. In one study common types of unhelpful support were:
  - minimising illness severity
  - pessimistic comments
  - pity or overly solicitous attitudes (Affleck et al. 1988).

Support needs change over time in response to changing treatment regime demands, disability, pain and symptomatology. What may be useful one day may be perceived as inappropriate the next.

Implications for clinical practice

Social support is amenable to change through psychosocial intervention. Goals for practitioners to work towards are:

- teaching patients how to develop and maintain family ties
- teaching patients how to recognise and accept the help and emotional encouragement provided by family members
- improving family members' skills for determining the patients' support needs, and offering help
- facilitating positive appraisals of support.

The key is to promote open communication among family members including feedback, and not criticism, when the help that was offered was not the help that was desired (Revenson 1990).

Spouses of chronically ill patients should be encouraged to build support networks outside the marriage, both within their existing social milieu and through more formal support groups of others facing similar stresses. These networks become critically important as the patients' health declines and disability increases, however, network building should be encouraged in the early stages of the illness so that networks are in place later on, when the patient is more limited and social activities with the support network may be restricted.

Depression in rheumatic disease

The onset of symptoms and eventual diagnosis of a chronic disease typically cause emotional distress. In most cases this distress subsides over time as psychological adaptation to the condition occurs (Rodin et al. 1991). A significant minority of people, however, will develop less transient and more severe psychological distress that can result in additional disability and suffering. Depression is the most common psychological disturbance associated with medical illness and can significantly increase the disability associated with the medical condition (Wells et al. 1989). Depression in the medically ill frequently goes undetected and untreated. If this is so the depression can become progressively debilitating and interfere with the optimal treatment for the medical condition. The presence of depression in rheumatic disease is particularly problematic, as it is often associated with somatic symptoms that overlap or resemble symptoms of arthritis. To further complicate the picture, depression can lead to the amplification of somatic symptoms of arthritis, causing physician and patient to mistakenly attribute worsening symptoms and disability to worsening of the medical condition. This in turn can result in unwarranted treatment changes and overmedication (Katon and Sullivan 1990). Depression is a debilitating and often life-threatening disorder and rheumatologists must be on the alert for depressive comorbidity among their patients and be prepared to provide appropriate treatment or referral. A diagnosis of major depression requires the occurrence of one or more major depressive episodes. A major depressive episode requires the presence of at least five of the following symptoms for at least two weeks:

- depressed mood
- diminished interest and pleasure in activities
- significant weight loss or gain
- sleep disturbance
- agitation or retardation
- fatigue or loss of energy
- feelings of worthlessness or guilt
- poor concentration
- recurrent thoughts of death or suicide.

One of the first two symptoms *must* be included in the five required to diagnose a depressive episode. Symptoms clearly due to a physical condition do not satisfy the diagnostic criteria, e.g. fatigue (American Psychiatric Association 1987). Most of the research efforts have focused on psychological sequelae in five rheumatological conditions (rheumatoid arthritis, juvenile rheumatoid arthritis, systemic lupus erythematosus, fibromyalgia and osteoarthritis) (Baum 1982). The majority of studies suggest that there is a greater prevalence of depressive symptoms and depressive disorders among clinical samples of people with rheumatological diseases than in the general population. The level of disturbance, however, is comparable to that found among clinical samples of people with other chronic medical conditions. Rheumatological disease severity and status have, at most, a very weak direct relation to the presence of depressive disorders and level of depressive symptoms. Depressive disorders and symptoms among people with rheumatological diseases are influenced more by pain, socioeconomic factors and social and other psychological resources, such as social support, a sense of control, illness intrusiveness and coping than by disease severity itself. Depressive disorders and even depressive symptoms have devastating effects on social, family and vocational functioning, and when added to a chronic medical condition, such as arthritis, functional declines are cumulative. Compared to the general population, the prevalence of depressive disorders and symptoms appear to be higher among people with rheumatological diseases. Rheumatologists therefore must be alert to depressive comorbidity and must guard against mistakenly attributing the additive effects of these comorbid conditions to worsening primary medical illness (DeVellis 1993).

References

Affleck G, Pfeiffer C, Tennen H, Fifield J (1988) Social support and psychosocial adjustment to rheumatoid arthritis. Arthritis Care and Research 1: 71–77.

American Psychiatric Association Committee on Nomenclature and Statistics (1987) Diagnostic and Statistical Manual of Mental Disorders Revised edn. (DSM-III-R). Washington DC: American Psychiatric Association 111–12, 213–33, 329–31.

Ansell BM (1977) Joint manifestations in children with juvenile chronic arthritis. Arthritis and Rheumatism 20: 204–6.

Arnett FC, Edworthy SM, Bloch DA et al. (1988) American Rheumatism Association 1987 revised criteria for the classification of rheumatoid arthritis. Arthritis and Rheumatism 31: 315–24.

Ashcroft J (1996) A patient's perspective. In Long AF, Scott DL (eds) Measuring Outcomes in Rheumatoid Arthritis. London: Royal College of Physicians. Ch 5: 29–34.

Ashcroft J (1997) Understanding people's everyday needs. Arthritis– getting it right – a guide for planners. London: Arthritis Care.

Baum J (1982) A review of the psychological aspects of rheumatic diseases. Seminars in Arthritis and Rheumatism 11: 352–61.

Bennet RM (1993) Psoriatic arthritis. In: McCarty DJ, Koopman WJ (eds) Arthritis and Allied Conditions – A Textbook of Rheumatology, 12th edn. Pennsylvania: Lea & Febiger. Ch 61 1079–94.

Bird HA, le Gallez P, Hill J (1985) Combined Care of the Rheumatic Patient. Berlin: Springer-Verlag.

Blocka KLN, Bassett LW, Furst DE, Clements PJ, Paulus HE (1981) The arthropathy of advanced progressive systemic sclerosis: a radiographic survey. Arthritis and Rheumatism 24: 874–84.

Burckhardt C (1985) The impact of arthritis on quality of life. Nursing Research 34: 11–16.

Carr AJ (1996) Measuring handicap. In Long AF, Scott DL (eds) Measuring Outcomes in Rheumatoid Arthritis. London: Royal College of Physicians. Ch 9: 61–70.

Cassidy JT (1994) Juvenile chronic arthritis. In: Klippel JH, Dieppe P (eds) Rheumatology. London: Mosby-Year Book Europe. 3: 20.1–20.10.

Cush JJ, Lipsky PE (1993) Reiter's syndrome and reactive arthritis. In: McCarty DJ, Koopman WJ (eds) Arthritis and Allied Conditions– A textbook of Rheumatology, 12th edn. Pennsylvania: Lea & Febiger. Ch 60: 1061–78.

DeVellis BM (1993) Depression in rheumatological diseases. In Newman S, Shipley M (eds) Psychological aspects of rheumatic diseases. Clinical Rheumatology. London: WB Saunders (Baillière Tindall) Ch 3: 241–57.

Dickey BF, Myers AR (1984) Pulmonary disease in polymyositis/dermatomyositis. Seminars in Arthritis and Rheumatism 14: 60–76.

Dieppe P, Doherty M, Macfarlane DG, Maddison PJ (1985) Rheumatological Medicine. Edinburgh: Churchill Livingstone.

Doherty M (1993) Fibromyalgia syndrome. Reports on rheumatic diseases Series 2 No. 23. Chesterfield: Arthritis and Rheumatism Council.

Doyle DV (1996) The rheumatologist's perspective. In: Long AF, Scott DL (eds) Measuring Outcomes in Rheumatoid Arthritis. London: Royal College of Physicians. Ch 4: 23–7.

Edwards J (1991) UCL Notes on Rheumatology. Sponsored by Roche Products Ltd. Broadwater, herts: Broadwater Press.

Ferrari R, Cash J, Maddison P (1996) Rheumatology Guidebook – A step-by-step guide to Diagnosis and Treatment. Oxford: BIOS.

Fitzpatrick R, Newman S, Lamb R, Shipley M (1988) Social relationships and psychological well-being in rheumatoid arthritis. Social Science and Medicine 27: 399–403.

Flor H, Turk DC, Scholz OB (1987) Impact of chronic pain on the spouse: marital, emotional and physical consequences. Journal of Psychosomatic Research 31: 63–71.

Gladman DD, Urowitz MB (1994) Systemic lupus erythematosus: clinical features. In: Klippel JH, Dieppe P (eds) Rheumatology. London: Mosby-Year Book Europe. 6: 2.1–18.

Goetz RH (1945) Pathology of progressive systemic sclerosis (generalized scleroderma) with special reference to changes in the viscera. Clinical Proceedings (Cape Town) 4: 337–42.

Gordon DA, Hastings DE (1994) Rheumatoid arthritis – clinical features: early, progressive and late disease. In Klippel JH, Dieppe P (eds) Rheumatology. London: Mosby-Year Book Europe. 3: 4.1–14.

Hawley DJ, Wolfe F (1988) Anxiety and depression in patients with rheumatoid arthritis: a prospective study of 400 patients. Journal of Rheumatology 15: 932–41.

Healey LA (1993) Polymyalgia and giant cell arteritis. In McCarty DJ, Koopman WJ (eds) Arthritis and allied conditions – A textbook of Rheumatology, 12th edn. Pennsylvania: Lea & Febiger. Ch 81: 1377–80.

Helliwell PS, Wright V (1994) Psoriatic arthritis: clinical features. In Klippel JH, Dieppe P (eds) Rheumatology. London: Mosby-Year Book Europe. 3: 31.1–8.

Hilliquin P, Menkes C-J (1994) Rheumatoid arthritis – evaluation and management. Early and established disease. In: Klippel JH, Dieppe P (eds) Rheumatology. London: Mosby-Year Book Europe. Section 3: 13.1–14.

Hirsch BJ, Moos RH, Reischl TM (1985) Psychosocial adjustment of adolescent children of a depressed, arthritic or normal parent. Journal of Abnormal Psychology 94: 154–64.

Hirsch BJ, Reischl TM (1985) Social networks and developmental psychopathology: a comparison of adolescent children of a depressed, arthritic or normal parent. Journal of Abnormal Psychology 94: 272–81.

Hughes RA (1996) Practical Problems – Septic Arthritis. Reports on Rheumatic Diseases Series 3 No. 7. London: Arthritis and Rheumatism Council for Research.

Judd M (1997) Caring for the patient with bone and joint disease. In Walsh M (Ed) Watson's Clinical Nursing and Related Sciences, 5th edn. London: Baillière Tindall. Ch 22: 873–98.

Katon W, Sullivan MD (1990) Depression and chronic medical illness. Journal of Clinical Psychiatry 51 (supplement): 3–14.

Keat A (1995) Reiter's Syndrome and Reactive Arthritis. Collected Reports on the Rheumatic Diseases. London: Arthritis and Rheumatism Council for Research. pp. 61–4.

Kellgren JH, Samuel EP (1950) The sensitivity and innervation of the articular capsule. Journal of Bone and Joint Surgery 32B: 84–92.

Kimberly RP, Urowitz MB (1994) Connective tissue disorders. In Klippel JH, Dieppe P (eds) Rheumatology. London: Mosby-Year Book Europe. 6: 1.1.

Leach M (1997) Juvenile chronic arthritis: epidemiology and genetics. Nursing Times 93(18): 46–8.

le Gallez P (1995) Rheumatoid arthritis. Primary Health Care 5(7): 31–8.

Leigh JP, Fries JF (1991) Education level and rheumatoid arthritis: evidence from five data centers. Journal of Rheumatology 18: 24–34.

Levine JD, Goetzl EJ, Basbaum AI (1987) Contribution of the nervous system to the pathophysiology of rheumatoid arthritis and other polyarthritides. Rheumatic Disease Clinics of North America 13: 369–83.

Long AF, Scott DL (1994) Measuring health status and outcomes in rheumatoid arthritis within routine clinical practice. British Journal of Rheumatology 33: 682–5.

Maini RN, Feldman M (1993) Immunopathogenesis of rheumatoid arthritis. In Maddison PJ et al. (eds) Oxford Textbook of Rheumatology. Volume 11. Oxford: Oxford University Press.

Manne SL, Zautra AJ (1989) Spouse criticism and support: their association with coping and psychological adjustment among women with rheumatoid arthritis. Journal of Personality and Social Psychology 56: 608–17.

Maricq HR (1981) Widefield capillary microscopy. Technique and rating scale for abnormalities seen in scleroderma and related disorders. Arthritis and Rheumatism 24: 1159–63.

Martin J, Meltzer H, Elliot D (1988) The prevalence of disability among adults. OPCS surveys of disability in Great Britain. Report 1. London: HMSO.

Matteson EL, Cohen MD, Conn DL (1994) Rheumatoid arthritis clinical features – systemic involvement. In: Klippel JH, Dieppe P (eds) Rheumatology. London: Mosby-Year Book Europe. 3: 5.1.

McClosky DA, Patella SJ, Seibold JR (1990) Health assessment questionnaire in systemic sclerosis. Proceedings of the Allied Health Professions 25th Meeting. p. 182.

McFarlane AC, Brooks PM (1988) Determinants of disability in rheumatoid arthritis. British Journal of Rheumatology 27: 7–14.

Medsger TA, Masi AT (1971) Epidemiology of systemic sclerosis (scleroderma). Annals of Internal Medicine 74: 714–21.

Medsger AR, Robinson H (1972) A comparative study of divorce in rheumatoid arthritis and other rheumatic diseases. Journal of Chronic Disease 25: 269–75.

Nicholas NS, Panayi GS (1988) Rheumatoid arthritis in pregnancy. Clinical and Experimental Rheumatology 6: 179–82.

Pisetsky DS (1994) Rheumatic disease etiology: immune-mediated inflammation. In Klippel JH, Dieppe P (eds) Rheumatology. London: Mosby-Year Book Europe. 1: 13.1–6.

Radojevic V, Nicassio PM, Weisman MH (1992) Behavioral intervention with and without family support for rheumatoid arthritis. Behavior Therapy 23: 13–30.

Revenson TA (1990) Social support processes among chronically ill elders: patient and provider perspectives. In: Giles H, Coupland N, Wiemann J (eds) Communication, Health and the Elderly. Manchester: Manchester University Press. pp. 92–113.

Revenson TA, Majerovitz SD (1990) Spouses' support provision to chronically ill patients. Journal of Social and Personal Relationships 7: 575–86.

Rodin G, Craven J, Littlefield C (1991) Depression in the medically ill: an integrated approach. New York: Brunner/Mazel. pp.1–91.

Rodnan GP, Benedek TG (1962) An historical account of the study of progressive systemic sclerosis (diffuse scleroderma). Annals of Internal Medicine 57: 305–19.

Ross AC (1990) Infection complicating orthopedic procedures and arthroplasties. Current Opinion in Rheumatology 2: 628–34.

Ryan S (1997) Rheumatology – knowledge for practice. Nursing Times Learning Curve 1(2): 5–8.

Schmid FR (1993) Principles of diagnosis and treatment of bone and joint infections. In McCarty DJ, Koopman WJ (eds) Arthritis and allied conditions – A textbook of Rheumatology, 12th edn. Pennsylvania: Lea & Febiger. Ch 115: 1975 –2001.

Schumacher HR, Schimmer B, Gordon GV et al. (1979) Articular manifestations of polymyositis and dermatomyositis. American Journal of Medicine 67: 287–92.

Segal R, Caspi D, Tisher M et al. (1988) Accelerated nodulosis and vasculitis during methotrexate therapy for RA. Arthritis and Rheumatism 31: 1182.

Simkin PA (1994) The musculoskeletal system. In: Klippel JH, Dieppe P (eds) Rheumatology. London: Mosby-Year Book Europe. 1: 2.1–2.10.

Solomon L, Robin G, Valkenburg HA (1975) Rheumatoid arthritis in an urban South African Negro population. Annals of the Rheumatic Diseases 34: 128–33.

Southwood T (1993) School children with arthritis. Head Teachers Review, Winter, 20–22.

Staines GL (1986) Men and women in role relationships. In Ashmore RD, Del Boca FK (eds) The Social Psychology of Female-Male Relations. New York: Academic Press. pp. 211–58.

Symmons D, Bankhead C (1994) Health care needs assessment for musculoskeletal diseases. London: Arthritis and Rheumatism Council for Research.

Symmons DPM, Jones M, Osborn J, Sills J, Southwood TR, Woo P (1996) Paediatric rheumatology in the United Kingdom: Data from the British Paediatric Rheumatology Group Register. British Journal of Rheumatology 23(11): 1975–80.

Varani J, Mulligan MS, Ward PA (1994) The vascular endothelium and acute inflammation. In Klippel JH, Dieppe P (eds) Rheumatology. London: Mosby-Year Book Europe. 3: 11.1–11.12.

Walker GL, Mastalgia FL, Roberts DF (1982) A search for genetic influence in idiopathic inflammatory myopathy. Acta Neurol Scand. 66: 432–3.

Weller BF (Ed) (1997) Ballière's Nurses' Dictionary, 22nd edn. London: Baillière Tindall p. 34.

Wells KB, Stewart A, Hays RD et al. (1989) The functioning and well-being of depressed patients: results from the Medical Outcomes Study. JAMA 262(7): 914–19.

White P (1994) Juvenile Chronic Arthritis – Clinical Features. In Klippel JH, Dieppe P (eds) Rheumatology. London: Mosby-Year Book Europe. 3: 17.1–17.10.

Wilske KR (1996) Rheumatoid arthritis: evolving concepts in therapy 'Don't fiddle while joints burn'. Rheumatology in Europe. EULAR 25(4): 145–9.

Wolfe F, Cathey MA (1991) The assessment and predication of functional disability in rheumatoid arthritis. Journal of Rheumatology 18: 1298–306.

Wolfe F, Hawley DJ, Cathey MA (1991) Clinical and health status measures over time: prognosis and outcome assessment in rheumatoid arthritis. Journal of Rheumatology 18: 1290–7.

Wood PNN (1971) Rheumatic complaints. British Medical Bulletin 27: 82–8.

WHO (1980) International Classification of Impairments, Disabilities and Handicaps (ICIDH), a manual of classification relating to the consequences of disease. Geneva: World Health Organisation.

WHO (1997) International Classification of Impairments, Activities, and Participation. (ICIDH–2), A Manual of Dimensions of Disablement and Functioning. Beta–1 draft for field trials. Geneva: World Health Organisation.

Part 2
Drug therapy

ANN BROWNFIELD AND SARAH RYAN

Objectives

After reading the chapters in Part 2 the reader should be able to:

*   explain the mechanism of pain
*   describe the purpose, mode of action and adverse effects of the major drug classifications used in the management of rheumatological conditions
*   discuss the drug management of a patient with inflammatory arthritis
*   debate the advantages and disadvantages of introducing a self-medication programme in the clinical area
*   discuss the role of complementary therapies in the management of arthritis.

2.1 Pain and its pharmacological management

The treatment of rheumatological disorders involves many components including education, exercise, adaptation and drug therapy. The main objectives of drug intervention are to:

- reduce or alleviate symptoms such as pain and stiffness
- suppress disease activity in chronic disorders such as rheumatoid arthritis.

This chapter provides the reader with an understanding of the purpose, mode of action, pharmacokinetics and adverse effects of the major drug classifications used in the management of rheumatological conditions. This will include:

- analgesia
- non-steroidal anti-inflammatory drug (NSAIDs)
- disease-modifying antirheumatic drugs (DMARDs)
- steroids.

Subsequent chapters will also explore the pharmacological management of gout, nursing innovations, e.g. self-medication and the role of complementary therapies in the care management of patients.

Drug therapy plays an important role in the management of inflammatory arthritis. It is hoped that these chapters will provide information on the wide ranging aspects of medications, enabling the nurse to share this knowledge with the patient so that a mutual understanding of care management can evolve.

The experience of pain can only be defined in terms of human consciousness. As with all sensory experience there is no way of being certain that one person's experience of pain is the same as another (Jones 1997). Pain is a paradox, being an accepted phenomena which is experienced by everyone at sometime during his or her life. It is also a unique, subjective and unverifiable personal experience (Turk and Melzack 1992). Pain is one of the cardial symptoms of rheumatoid arthritis and affects both physical and psychological aspects of functioning. It is the major contributor to the morbidity, disability and socioeconomic cost of muscloskeletal disorders (Cohen 1994).

Treatment interventions in the management of pain include:

- opioid drugs
- non-opioid and adjuvant analgesic drugs
- physical programmes
- cognitive and behavioural approaches (Cohen 1994).

Acute pain is a transient experience where the source of pain is usually identifiable. Here pharmacological interventions are able to suppress the pain stimuli (Pearce and Wardle 1989). In contrast, chronic pain is an ongoing experience; often patients may demonstrate an array of associated disorders such as anxiety depression and insomnia.

Within the realms of nursing the successful pharmacological control of pain dictates that nurses possess a comprehensive research-based pharmacological knowledge and effective interpersonal skills to enable the assessment, planning, implementation and evaluation of pharmacological interventions in the management of pain (Lubkin 1990).

Physiology of pain

The gate control theory

The gate control theory originates from Melzack and Wall (1982). It has been most influential in developing our present understanding of the mechanism of pain. Occasionally viewed as oversimplified or too rigid it has provided a framework which demonstrated the complexity of the pain response (Jackson 1995).

The theory is founded on two main concepts (see Figure 2.1):

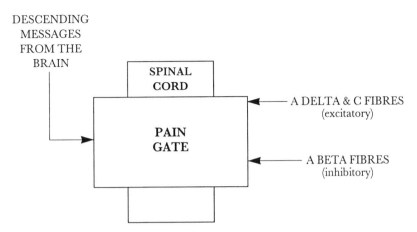

Figure 2.1 Influences on the pain gate

- The transmission of pain messages can be modulated within the spinal cord. This occurs via descending messages from the brain which inhibits sensations from peripheral and internal sources being experienced as pain. Two neurotransmitters appear to be involved in this process. The release of *enkephalin* at the spinal cord inhibits the uptake of calcium ions by the spinal cord neurones. This prevents further transmission of the pain message. *Serotonin* (the second neurotransmitter) is involved in the transmission of pain messages between the raphe magnus and the cord.
- The transmission of pain messages to the brain can be altered by activating another source of sensory receptor. When pain impulses enter the dorsal horn of the spinal cord the gate control mechanism is either opened or closed. A number of laminae within the dorsal horn forms the gate control mechanism and this specialised area enabled the pain impulses to be modulated (Jackson 1995).

The primary sensory neurones involved in pain transmission are:

- *Type A delta fibres:* small myelinated fibres capable of transporting messages at speeds of 6–30 m/second.
- *Type C fibres:* very small, with no myelin insulation, so messages are transmitted a lot slower at speeds of 0.5–2 m/second (Guyton 1991). Type C fibres transmit slower chronic pain.
- *Type A beta fibres:* are larger fibres than other sensory neurones and electrical impulses travel along them at a greater speed. Therefore, the pain stimulus conducted along type A(beta) fibres is quicker and faster than the transmission of the other fibres.

Impulses from Aα and C fibres are excitatory in nature and promote the release of an exitory neurotransmitter, *substance P*, which *opens* the gate facilitating the perception of pain. The opening of the gate allows the transmission of pain impulses along the spinoreticular and reticular thalamic tracts through various junctions into the sensory cortex (Fordham 1986). If activated, type Aα fibres occupy the secondary neurones first, thereby blocking other pain messages. These fibres can be activated by rubbing or vibration of the skin, and their activation *closes* the pain gate. This theory has been instrumental in the development of treatment interventions such as transcutaneous electrical nerve stimulation machines (TENS).

Studies of the thalamus and somatosensory cortex show that in arthritis some cells have an abnormally large response to joint stimulation, causing changes in the way impulses are transmitted (Newman et al. 1996).

Pain receptors

Sensory receptors are situated in the tissues of the body, especially in the skin, synovium of joints and walls of arteries. These receptors are referred to as *nociceptors* as they respond to noxious stimuli. Such receptors can be divided into three categories:

- *Mechanical changes:* in active inflammatory conditions such as rheumatoid arthritis, increased synovial fluid in the joint cavity and proliferation of the inflamed synovial tissues causes pain by distension and stretching of the capsule.
- *Temperature changes:* exposure of the tissues to extremes of temperature can cause stimulation of the receptors.
- *Inflammatory changes:* the inflammatory response initiated by tissue damage causes the release of prostaglandin, bradykinin, histamine and serotonin. This stimulates a reaction in the receptors.

Some nociceptor receptors respond to all the above stimulants. They terminate in the dorsal horn of the spinal cord and transmit their pain messages to secondary neurones. The destination for secondary neurones is the thalamus.

Role of the brain

Pain signals terminate in the brain. Fast pain signals are relayed via the brain stem and the thalamus to areas of the cortex, especially the somatosensory area. This region of the cortex can differentiate the area of the origin of the pain message.

Slow pain messages are relayed over a wide area of the brain stem and thalamus. The reticuloactivating system is situated in the brain stem; when it is stimulated it increases the excitability of the brain. This is why people with chronic pain conditions such as fibromyalgia report difficulty in sleeping, resting and relaxing. It also explains why chronic pain is difficult to locate, because the pain messages are not relayed to the somatosensory areas.

Once stimulation of the receptor ceases so should the pain; but pain pathways cannot explain all pain experiences and patients can continue to experience pain after its original cause has been removed. Woolf (1994) offers a theory for the development of chronic pain states. He proposes that neurones in the dorsal horn of the spinal cord become hypersensitive and develop alternative synapses with neighbouring neurones. This causes pain messages to go astray.

Also, other substances released within the spinal cord can mediate the transmission of pain signals. N-Methyl-d-aspartate (NMDA) and neurokinin (NK) cause the spinal cord neurones to become hypersensitive. This can cause the phenomena of *hyperalgesia* (severe pain to a stimuli that would normally only produce mild pain) or *allodynia* (pain in response to a stimulus that would not normally be painful, such as stroking the skin (Woolf 1994).

Additionally, many aspects of higher levels of processing have a considerable effect on how unpleasant a pain stimulus is. The experience of pain is influenced by anxiety, cultural factors, the environment and past experiences (Gibson 1994). Reassurances that a stimulus will be brief considerably reduces the unpleasantness rating (Jones 1997).

This assumes that there is an inevitable behavioural sequence that is initiated by a noxious stimulant, referred to as the 'bottom up approach' (Jones 1997). However, the brain is quite capable of simply ignoring noxious stimulus altogether under conditions of severe stress (Melzack and Wall 1982) and it is capable of selecting what sensory information is acted on; this is known as the 'top down approach'. It is the balance between these ascending and descending processes that determine our perception of pain (Jones 1997).

Physiological effects of acute pain

Once the acute pain impulse has passed the gate control mechanism it enters the reticular activating system and sympathetic nervous system activity increases, aiding the body's flight or fight mechanism (Jordan 1992).

This activity includes:

- an increase in *hormonal activity*:
  - *antidiuretic hormone* increases the reabsorption from the renal tubules retaining water within the body (this can elevate blood pressure)
  - *aldosterone* increases the reasorption of sodium from the renal tubules
  - *adrenaline* causes increased consciousness and emotion
  - *cortisol* increases blood glucose levels and the secretion of hydrochloric acid and pepsinogen
- an increase in *cardiovascular activity*; tachycardia and increased cardiac output.
- an increase in *gastric activity* leading to a reduction in gastric emptying.

2.2 Pharmacological interventions in rheumatology

The major pharmacological interventions for the management of pain include the following categories of drug therapy:

* non-opioid analgesia
* compound analgesia
* opioid analgesia
* antidepressant drugs
* non-steroidal anti-inflammatory drugs (NSAIDs).

Non-opioid analgesia

Non-opioid analgesics are administered to treat mild to moderate pain. Ranked by clinical efficacy, they represent the first rung on the analgesic ladder.

Acetaminophen – paracetamol

Paracetamol is an undervalued effective analgesic agent (Cohen 1994). Its mechanism of action remains poorly understood, although there is evidence of direct effect on the central nervous system (CNS) rather than on peripheral tissue. It blocks the synthesis and secretion of prostaglandin, preventing nociceptor sensitization (Speight 1987). It has both analgesic and antipyretic properties.

Pharmacokinetics

Taken orally, paracetamol is well absorbed from the gastrointestinal tract and inactivated in the liver. A major advantage is the lack of upper gastrointestinal toxicity, especially ulceration and bleeding.

Adverse effects

The well-known hazard of hepatoxicity is virtually only seen in conjunction with a drug overdose and is increased with liver disease and alcoholism. The daily dose should be closely monitored in these situations. The risk of nephrotoxicity with chronic dosing remains uncertain but is probably very small (Cohen 1994).

NEFOPAM HYDROCHLORIDE (ACUPAN)

Nefopam provides strong and rapid relief for moderate to severe pain that has not been alleviated with other non-narcotic analgesia (Walker 1994). Its mode of action of is not fully understood. It is known to act on the CNS and it has the ability to alter pain perception within the brain. Nefopam does not cause respiratory depression or addiction, but it does possess anticholinergic and sympathomimetic actions which are responsible for some of the common side effects, e.g. nervousness, dry mouth and nausea.

Compound analgesia

Compound analgesics are fixed ratio combinations of non-opioid (aspirin or paracetamol) and opioid analgesia (dextropropoxyphene or codeine preparations).

Compound analgesics contain either a low dose or full dose of opioid analgesic and can thus bridge the therapeutic gap between non-opioid and opioid analgesia. However, it is worth noting that the compound or combined analgesic effect may also result in a combination of the side effects of both types of analgesia. Examples of these

Table 2.1 Adverse effects of compound analgesia

Dizziness
Sedation
Nausea/vomiting
Constipation
Abdominal pain
Rashes
Headaches
Weakness
Euphoria
Dysphoria
Hallucinations
Minor visual disturbances
Abnormal liver function tests

drugs include co-codamol, co-dydramol, co-codaprin and co-prox-amol. Adverse effects are shown in Table 2.1.

Opioids

Severe pain may require opioid analgesics. These drugs are classified in terms of their efficacy as low or high efficacy opioids (see Table 2.2). Their role in the management of moderate to severe musculoskeletal pain is controversial (Cohen 1994). Although certain patients may benefit without experiencing adverse effects and addiction, the question of true efficacy has not yet been answered (Jamison 1996).

Table 2.2 Opioids

Low efficacy	High efficacy
Codeine	Buprenorphine
Dihydrocodeine	Dextromaramide
Dextropropoxyphene	Diamorphine
Nalbuphine	Dipipanone
Pentazocine	Meptazinal
	Methadone
	Morphine
	Papaveretum
	Pethidine
	Tramadol

Opioid analgesics work by fitting into the opioid receptors of the brain and spinal cord. These receptors are also used by endorphins, the body's own opioid. Opioid analgesia inhibits the transmission of nociceptive messages to the higher centres or through activation of the descending antinociceptive pathways (Ferrante 1983). Evidence from Stein (1991) highlights the peripheral analgesic action of these medications in conditions characterised by inflammatory hyperalgesia.

Low efficacy opioids

CODEINE PHOSPHATE

Primarily prescribed as an analgesic but also used as an antidiarrhoea drug and a cough suppressant, codeine has been in use for nearly 100 years. Although codeine's analgesic properties are similar to those of morphine its analgesic action is only approximately 10% as powerful.

Pharmacokinetics

Taken orally, codeine is quickly absorbed within the gastrointestinal tract and metabolised within the liver. It has a half-life of approximately 2–3 hours. Excretion is via the kidneys into the urine. The analgesic effect of 30 mg of codeine is suggested to equal that of 300–600 mg of apririn.

DIHYDROCODEINE TARTRATE

Dihydrocodeine has a similar analgesic effect to codeine.

DEXTROPROPOXYPHENE HYDROCHLORIDE

The analgesic effect of dextropropoxyphene is considerably less than that of codeine. Chemically it is structurally related to methadone but it possesses less analgesic, antitussive and dependency properties. Its main use is as a compound analgesic either with paracetamol (co-proxamol) or with aspirin (doloxene).

Pharmacokinetics

Dextropropoxyphene is rapidly absorbed in the gastrointestinal tract and metabolised within the liver. In the event of an overdose the rapid absorption of this drug can produce respiratory arrest, hypotension and cardiac dysrhythmia within one hour.

High efficacy opioids

BUPRENORPHINE (TEMGESIC)

Buprenorphine can be useful because of the length (6 hours) and strength of its analgesic properties. It also possesses both opioid agonist and antagonist qualities and is therefore less likely to produce addiction, respiratory depression or affect cardiovascular function than other opioid analgesics.

Pharmacokinetics

Administered sublingually because of presystemic elimination.

DEXTROMORAMIDE (PALFIUM)

A derivative of the opium poppy, dextromoramide is a powerful quick-acting analgesic which has been prescribed in the UK since the 1950s for severe and intractable pain. It has a shorter duration of action than morphine, and is less sedating. It can therefore produce pain relief without affecting consciousness or mental activity or inducing constipation, unlike other opioids.

Concominant administration of tranquillisers such as chlorpromazine produces a synergistic analgesic effect.

Pharmacokinetics

Taken orally, dextromoramide is quickly absorbed and metabolised within the liver. It is short acting, with a duration of approximately 3 hours.

DIAMORPHINE HYDROCHLORIDE

Introduced a century ago, diamorphine is indicated for both severe and chronic pain. It is a powerful opioid analgesic which is a derivative of the unripe seed pod of the opium poppy. Although diamorphine mirrors morphine in its actions and uses, it can produce enhanced pain relief with fewer adverse effects such as nausea or hypotension.

Pharmacokinetics

Following administration, diamorphine is rapidly converted into monoacetyl morphine and more slowly metabolised into its main active metabolite, morphine. Within 24 hours approximately 80% of the dose is excreted via the urine.

FENTANYL

Fentanyl is more efficacious than morphine. It is normally administered as an intraoperative analgesic. More recently it has been introduced for chronic pain in the form of a patch for transdermal drug delivery (Durogesic). This mode of administration can maintain its efficacy for 72 hours.

MORPHINE

Derived from the opium and in use since the nineteenth century, morphine is prescribed for moderate to severe pain in both acute and chronic conditions. It acts on the CNS to eliminate pain and can also transform the unpleasant sensation of pain into a sense of euphoria. Morphine therefore has two major effects, one depressing, the other stimulating (Trouce and Gould 1990). The 'depressing' effects of morphine can include:

- Reduction of the appreciation of pain.
- Suppression of respiration and the cough reflex.
- Reduction of anxiety and the feeling of euphoria.
- Some level of sedation (owing to its mildly hypnotic properties).
- Reduction of the peristaltic activities of the bowel.
- Urinary retention.

The stimulant effects of morphine can include:

- Increased arousal of the chemoreceptor trigger zone within the brain stem including nausea and vomiting.
- Increased arousal of the vagus nerve which may produce such effects as bradycardia and hypotension, owing to a parasympathic action in the cardiovascular system (Trouce and Gould 1990).

Morphine works on specific opioid receptors situated throughout the body. Such receptors are divided into categories and include delta (α), kappa (κ), and mu (μ) receptors. It is the mu receptor on which morphine has its main effects. Mu receptors are associated with analgesia, respiratory depression, euphoria and dependence (Walker 1994). The pharmacological effects of morphine on each individual can differ considerably (Rowbotham 1993).

Pharmacokinetics

Following oral administration, morphine is absorbed from the gastrointestinal tract where it undergoes conjugation in the gut wall and liver, with approximately 20% of the dose actually reaching the systemic circulation. Elimination of most morphine is via the kidneys in the urine. Subcutaneous and intramuscular administration is quicker than oral administration. The drug interactions and adverse effects are shown in Tables 2.3 and 2.4 respectively.

Table 2.3 Drug interactions of opioids

Alcohol	enhances the sedative and hypotensive effects
Antidepressants	may result in CNS excitement or depression
Antipsychotics	enhance the sedative and hypotensive effects
Anxiolytics and hypnotics	enhance the sedative effects
Antihistamines	enhances the sedative effects
Cisparide	may antagonise the effect of gastrointestinal motility
Ulcer healing drugs	increase plasma concentrations of opioids
Antiemetics	antagonise the effects of gastrointestinal activity

Table 2.4 Adverse effects of opioids

Nausea and vomiting
Constipation
Respiratory depression
Hypotension
Dry mouth
Micturition difficulties
Bradycardia/tachycardia
Hallucinations
Mood changes
Addiction
Reduced libido

PETHIDINE HYDROCHLORIDE

Akin to morphine, pethidine provides rapid pain relief for short periods of time. Prescribed inappropriately it can be addictive.

TRAMADOL HYDROCHLORIDE (ZYDOL)

Tramadol can enhance both serotonenergic and adrenergic pathways. It is considered the equal of morphine in terms of its efficacy when prescribed for moderate chronic pain, but is less likely than morphine to cause respiratory depression, addiction or constipation.

Pharmacokinetics

Administered orally, tramadol is quickly absorbed from the gastrointestinal tract. It possesses a half-life of 6 hours. It is excreted in the urine and approximately a third of the dose is excreted unchanged.

Antidepressants

Antidepressant therapy may enhance the analgesic effect induced by other drugs. The presumed site of action is at the spinal cord level. Although there is beneficial effect on sleep and mood, suggesting action elsewhere in the neuroaxis, debate continues over possible modes of action and whether or not these drugs induce analgesia in the absence of depression in chronic pain generally (Watson 1994).

Tricyclic drugs

The increased incidence of anxiety and depression amongst chronic pain sufferers is not the only justification put forward for the use of tricyclic drugs. They also appear to have a synergistic effect with centrally acting analgesia and the stimulation of endorphin production (Brown and Bottomley 1990).

Non-steroidal anti-inflammatory drugs (NSAIDs)

NSAIDs have become an integral part of the management of inflammatory conditions. The ultimate goal of NSAID therapy is to reduce inflammation. The decision to commence therapy includes consideration of the risks weighted against the potential for therapeutic benefit for the patient and should take into account the nature of the underlying condition and the severity of the patient's symptoms.

The objective of commencing NSAIDs is to decrease the cardinal symptoms of inflammation which include pain, stiffness, swelling and warmth. These symptoms are not only unpleasant for the patient but also affect physical and psychological functioning. In addition to reducing inflammation this group of drugs also possesses analgesic and antipyretic properties which are necessary to treat the associated features of inflammation. The effectiveness of NSAID should be evident within a few days and they make an almost immediate impression on the patient's symptoms. The therapy will continue to be effective as long as blood levels of the drug are maintained. Stopping this therapy for any reason could result in a recurrence of the symptoms of inflammation.

Although the patient will start to feel better once the features of inflammation are reduced, NSAID therapy does not influence the progression of conditions such as rheumatoid arthritis. In this situation a combined approach is required, often including the administration of an analgesic as well as a second-line drug such as methotrexate to suppress the disease activity.

Classification

The NSAIDs can be classified on the basis of their chemical structure. The older NSAIDs, e.g. indomethacin, have excellent anti-inflammatory properties but commonly produce adverse side effects especially on the gastrointestinal system, whereas agents such as the

propionic acid derivatives have less likelihood of causing side effects
and are generally better tolerated.

The chemical classification of the NSAIDs is shown in Table 2.5.

Table 2.5 Chemical classification of NSAIDs

Type of NSAID	Examples
Carboxylic acids	
Acetylated	Aspirin
Non-acetylated	Choline, salicylate, diflunisal
Acetic acids	Indomethacin, diclofenac, sulindac, etodaloc
Propionic acids	buprofen, flurbiprofen, fenbufen, fenoprofen, ketoprofen, tiaprofenic acid
Fenamic acids	Piroxicam, phenylbutazone, azapropazone, tenoxicam
Non-acidic compounds	Nabumetone
Cox-2 Inhibitor	Meloxicam

Which NSAID to use?

The choice between the various NSAIDs is largely empirical (Schlegel
1987). Huskisson et al. (1974) first demonstrated marked individual variability of response to NSAIDs in rheumatoid arthritis. The cause for
these differences is not known. If a patient experiences a poor response
to one NSAID, another should be tried. There can be a variation in
response even when the NSAID is from the same chemical family. Once
a NSAID is commenced the patient should be maintained on it for
2 weeks before an assessment of its efficacy is made, unless the patient
experiences an adverse reaction which would necessitate immediate
revision of the treatment. The ultimate goal of NSAID intervention is to
choose a preparation that combines the greatest effectiveness with the
least toxicity for each individual patient (Schlegel 1987).

Some NSAIDs are particularly useful in certain clinical situations.

- *Indomethacin* has been noted for its effect on the management of
  ankylosing spondylitis and gout.
- *Sulindac* is reported to have a renal sparing effect and may be the
  drug of choice in patients with impaired function (Thompson and
  Dunne 1995).

NSAIDs can be divided into two groups according to their half-life.
Those drugs with a half-life of greater than 12 hours, e.g. piroxicam,
tenoxicam and azapropazone, need only be administered once or

twice daily, which should aid compliancy. However, it should be noted that medications with a long half-life may build up excessively in the plasma of older patients, increasing the potential for the occurrence of side effects. The majority of other NSAIDs are referred to as short half-life drugs, as their half-life is usually less than 6 hours.

Administration

NSAIDs can be administered in many different ways: orally, as slow release compounds, intramuscularly, topically and in suppository form.

*   *Topical preparations* are available for only a few NSAIDs. They are more efficacious than placebo (Thompson and Dunne 1995). Local skin sensitivity may occur and there is some absorption into the circulation leading to the rare occurrence of systemic side effects.
*   *Suppositories* are useful to reduce the risk of gastric irritation by the direct effect of the drug on the mucosa. However, there is still a risk of gastric ulceration mediated via the circulation. NSAIDs given in suppository form can also cause local irritation in the rectum. Patients can also find them difficult to administer, especially if they have reduced manual dexterity.

Contra-indication: peptic ulcers

In patients with peptic ulcer disease NSAIDs are contra-indicated. If a patient has a history of peptic ulcer symptoms the clinician may well consider providing gastric cytoprotection. This may include the prescribing of H_2 receptor antagonists for duodenal ulcers and prostaglandin analogues for patients with gastric ulceration (Thompson and Dunne 1995). Proton pump inhibitors may also be considered as a different treatment option, e.g. omeprazole and lansoprazole. These drugs inhibit the gastric acid by blocking the hydrogen–potassium adenosine triphosphatase enzyme system (the proton pump) of the gastric parietal cell. They are the treatment of choice for stricturing and erosive oesophagitis and are effective in the short term treatments of gastric and duodenal ulcers.

Patients with a history of ulceration may also be prescribed a COX-2 inhibitor (e.g. meloxicam). Some health authorities recommend concurrent treatment in patients over the age of 65 or for those taking corticosteroid therapy in whom the risk of serious adverse gastrointestinal side effects is high.

Indicators for the use of NSAIDs

In chronic inflammatory rheumatology conditions such as rheumatoid arthritis, ankylosing spondylitis, psoriatic arthritis and connective tissue disorders (with polyarthritis) patients may well have to take NSAIDs on a regular basis to provide symptomatic relief from the effects of ongoing inflammation. If the patient experiences a reduction in disease activity they may no longer need regular administration of the NSAID therapy and a trial will establish whether this is the case. Because of the side effects that this group of drugs can cause, the safety of the overall treatment increases if the patient does not need the intervention.

Patients with osteoarthritis are often better managed on simple analgesia. In older patients the risk of side effects can outweigh the potential therapeutic effects of NSAIDs, although their use may be considered if the condition initiates a flare of inflammatory symptoms. Here the use of NSAIDs would be considered short term for symptom relief. Other conditions where it may be appropriate to use NSAIDs on a short term basis include gout, pseudogout and certain sport injuries.

Mode of action

NSAIDs appear to be involved in many of the pathways that are influential in the production of inflammatory mediators as well as actively involved in the interactions between inflammatory cells. NSAIDs are known to play a role in the suppression of prostaglandin synthesis partly by inhibiting the enzyme prostaglandin synthetase H (also known as cyclooxygenase, COX). Prostaglandins are synthesised from membrane phospholipids; when induced, they act to produce many of the features of inflammation including warmth, erythema and odema.

NSAIDs have effects on various other aspects of the inflammatory response including leukotriene synthesis, superoxide production and cytokine production (see Figure 2.2).

The suppression of prostaglandins by NSAIDs may help relieve the symptoms of inflammation but this suppression is also responsible for the major adverse effects of NSAIDs including gastrointestinal disturbances and effects on kidney functioning (Brooks 1994, Flowers 1996).

There is considerable interest in the discovery of the presence of different forms (isoforms) of the enzyme cox. Cox-1 is a constitutive

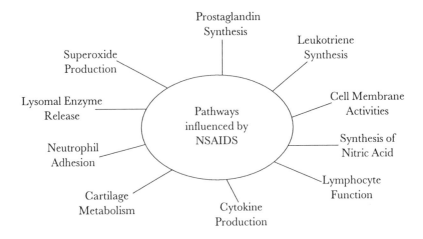

Figure 2.2 Pathways influenced by NSAIDs.

form of enzyme, i.e. it has a 'housekeeping' role in the normal cell in that it maintains the integrity of the gastric and duodenal mucosa and regulates renal blood flow. Cox-2 is produced in states of inflammation. Drugs now being marketed, e.g. meloxicam, claim to inhibit Cox-2 (to reduce inflammation) but do not inhibit the properties of Cox-1, thereby in theory reducing the likelihood of adverse effects occurring.

Pharmacokinetics

Most NSAIDs are completely absorbed from the gastrointestinal tract. They bind strongly to plasma proteins and are predominately cleared by the liver. The metabolites are excreted in the urine. Some NSAIDs are absorbed in the active form whereas others, referred to as *pro-drugs*, are converted by hepatic metabolism to active drugs.

Side effects

In general the NSAIDs share a common spectrum of side effects although the frequency of particular side effects varies between different compounds. Mild adverse effects are relatively common, occurring in approximately 10–15% of users. Because these drugs are prescribed in large numbers worldwide, a significant number of people experience more serious side effects. The major side effects occur in several organ systems. These include:

- gastrointestinal tract
- central nervous system
- haematopoetic system
- kidney
- skin
- liver.

Gastrointestinal tract

The gastrointestinal tract is the system most commonly affected by NSAIDs, often necessitating discontinuation of therapy. Symptoms patients may experience include dyspepsia, epigastric pain, indigestion, nausea and vomiting. Gastrointestinal lesions may range from hyperaemia to diffuse gastritis, erosions or ulcers.

Factors associated with increased risk of ulceration include:

- age (over 65 years)
- previous peptic ulcer disease
- concomitant steroid therapy
- heart failure
- high dose NSAIDs.

Low dose ibuprofen appears to be associated with a low risk of upper gastrointestinal symptoms. Diclofenac, naproxen and indomethacin are associated with intermediate risk of adverse events and azapropazone is associated with the highest risk. If patients experience adverse reactions it is necessary to carry out an endoscopy to assess any irritation or ulceration in the tract. All patients are advised to take NSAIDs with food.

Kidney

The synthesis of renal prostaglandins is simulated by vasoconstrictor substances involved in circulating haemostasis such as angiotensin II, noradrenaline and vasopressin. By modulating the effects of these vasoconstrictor substances on the kidney vasodilatory prostoglandin – especially prostaglandin E_2 and prostacyclin – help to maintain adequate renal blood flow and glomerular filtration rate. This modulatory effect plays a minor role in controlling renal function in healthy individuals but under circumstances of circulatory stress the prostaglandins become essential to the maintenance of adaquate renal function. In this situation, treatment with COX inhibitors such as NSAIDs may precipitate acute renal failure.

Risk factors for NSAID induced renal insufficiency include:

* congestive heart failure
* cirrhosis with ascites
* nephrotic syndrome
* age (over 60 years)
* concurrent diuretic therapy (which causes potassium retention).

Renal side effects from NSAIDs appear to be dose related and occur more often in elderly people (Thompson and Dunne 1995). NSAIDs can also affect the salt and water balance causing sodium retention which may result in hypertension, oedema or heart failure in predisposed individuals.

Drugs such as tiaprofenic acid have also been associated with cystitis. Acute interstitial nephritis and nephrotic syndrome has been linked with naproxen, indomethacin, phenylbutazone, fenoprofen and diflunisal. The pathogenesis is unknown.

Hypersensitivity phenomena may also be present with nephrotic syndrome including fever, skin rash and eosinophilia.

Central nervous system

Cognitive dysfunction, memory loss, inability to concentrate, confusion, personality change, forgetfulness, depression, sleeplessness and paranoid thoughts have all been reported in elderly patients treated with naproxen and ibuprofen (Goodwin and Regan 1982).

Headaches and dizziness may occur with indomethacin. Aspirin can affect hearing and cause tinnitus.

Several of the NSAIDs have been associated with aseptic meningitis, e.g. ibuprofen and sulindac (Schlegel 1987). Patients with collagen diseases seem to be at the highest risk from the complication.

Haematological reactions

The most common reaction is iron deficiency anaemia as a result of gastrointestinal blood loss that occurs secondary to erosion or ulceration. Blood dyscracias associated with NSAID therapy are rare, but among the major cause of death with this therapy. Agranulocytosis, thrombocytopenia, neutropenia and aplastic anaemia have all been reported. The latter is very rare except with phenylbutazone, the administration of which in the UK is limited to hospital prescriptions.

Inhibitors of platelet aggregation by NSAIDs may cause a mild prolongation of the bleeding time in patients. This becomes a particular concern for those patients receiving anticoagulation therapy or those who have hereditary clotting factor deficiencies.

Liver

NSAIDs can cause a transient rise in liver enzymes and, more rarely, a hepatic illness such as hepatitis. Patients of advanced age, with a reduced renal function and receiving high dose NSAID therapy, are at greatest risk of adverse liver reactions.

Respiratory system

NSAIDs may precipitate asthmatic attacks in predisposed individuals. In some patients with bronchial asthma the inhibition of COX may reduce bronchodilatory prostaglandins. This diverts arachidonic acid metabolism towards lipoxygenase products (leukotrienes). This activity may precipitate bronchospasm.

Pulmonary effects including effusions have been reported with ibuprofen, naproxen and phenylbutazone therapy.

Skin

All NSAIDs can provoke skin reactions including photosensitivity, vesiculobullous eruptions, serum sickness and exfoliative erythroderma. Urticaria has been reported with aspirin, ibuprofen and indomethacin.

Phenylbutazone and oxyphenbutazone are the NSAIDs that have the highest incidence of serious or fatal skin reactions including erythema multiforme, exofoliative dermatitis, Stevens–Johnson syndrome and toxic epidermal reaction.

Cutaneous vasculitis is a rare occurrence but has been related to the use of indomethacin, fenbufen and naproxen.

Pregnancy

The inhibitor of prostaglandin synthesis by NSAIDs during pregnancy may cause prolongation of gestation and increase postpartum and neonatal bleeding. NSAIDs should be avoided during pregnancy, especially as they may promote premature closure of the ductus arteriosus and impair fetal circulation.

Drug interactions

The major interactions that occur with the administration of NSAIDs are shown below. For safe practice, consult the manufacturer's guidelines before advocating usage.

- *Anticoagulant therapy:* may be enhanced.
- *Antidepressant therapy:* e.g. moclobemide, can acclerate the absorption of NSAIDS.
- *Cardioglycosides:* the plasma concentration of cardiac glycoside can be increased exacerbating heart failure.
- *Diuretics:* there is an increased risk of nephrotoxicity and a possible risk of hyperkalaemia associated with potassium-sparing diuretics.
- *Lithium:* there is an increased risk of toxicity.
- *Muscle relaxants:* (e.g.) baclofen, there is an increased risk of toxicity.
- *Ace inhibitors:* there is an increased risk of renal damage and an antagonistic hypotensive effect.
- *Beta-blockers:* NSAIDS are antagonistic of hypotensive effects.
- *Cytotoxic agents.* there is a reduction in the excretion of these agents. The potential interaction between NSAIDS and low dose methotrexate is not a problem at the dose used in patients with rheumatoid arthritis (Thompson and Dunne 1995).
- *Uricosurics*, e.g. probenecid: These drugs increase the plasma concentration of many NSAIDS and delay their excretion.
- *Antiepileptic drugs:* may be enhanced.

Interactions with specific NSAIDs

- *Brufen:* can increase digoxin levels.
- *Fenoprofen:* half-life may be reduced following the co-administration of barbiturates, e.g. phenobarbitone.
- *Ketoprofen:* may increase the level of sulphonamides in the blood.
- *Indomethacin:* increases the bioavailability of biophosphates.
- *Azapropazone:* may interfere with the action of oral hypoglycaemic drugs. Also the plasma concentration of azapropazone may increase with the administration of cimetidine.

The administration of two or more NSAIDs will increase the risk of adverse effects occurring.

Propionic acids

IBUPROFEN (BRUFEN, FENBID)

Ibuprofen possesses anti-inflammatory, analgesic and antipyretic properties. Its anti-inflammatory properties are weaker than those of other NSAIDs, so it potentially has fewer side effects.

Treatment regime

- *Adults:* orally with food 1.2–1.8 g daily in divided doses (maximum dose 2.4 g daily if required) taken with food.
- *Children:* 20 mg/kg daily in divided doses increasing up to 40 mg/kg in juvenile arthritis (not recommended for children weighing below 7 kg).

FENBUFEN

Fenbufen is both a NSAID and a non-narcotic analgesic which possesses a similar action to that of aspirin. It has been prescribed for the symptomatic relief of various musculoskeletal disorders. Although fenbufen has been associated with an increased risk of skin rashes it possesses a decreased risk of gastrointestinal bleeding.

Treatment regimes

- *Adults:* orally with food 300 mg in the morning and 600 mg at night or 450 mg twice daily. It is not recommended for children below 14 years of age.

FENOPROFEN

Fenoprofen is also a NSAID and a non-narcotic analgesic with properties akin to aspirin. Therapeutically it is considered to be as effective as naproxen and in comparison with ibuprofen it possesses a slightly higher risk of gastrointestinal disturbances.

Treatment regimes

- *Adults:* orally with food 200–600 mg in 3–4 divided doses – not more than 3 g daily.
- *children:* not recommended.

FLURBIPROFEN

Flurbiprofen is both an anti-inflammatory and a non-narcotic analgesic with effects similar to aspirin. It is considered more effective therapeutically than naproxen, but has a greater potential for gastrointestinal disturbances than ibuprofen.

Treatment regimes
- *Adults:* orally or rectally 150–200 mg daily, increasing to a maximum of 300 mg daily for acute conditions.
- *Children:* not recommended.

KETOPROFEN

Ketoprofen possesses anti-inflammatory and analgesic properties: therapeutically it is considered akin to ibuprofen, but potentially it has more side effects.

Treatment regimes
- *Adults:*
  - orally with food 100–200 mg daily in divided doses.
  - rectally 100 mg at night.
  - combined prescriptions of oral and rectal preparations should not exceed 200 mg daily.
  - deep intramuscular injection 50–100 mg 3–4 hourly: total dose not to exceed 200 mg in 24 hours.

NAPROXEN

Naproxen has anti-inflammatory, analgesic and antipyretic properties.

Treatment regimes
- *Adults:*
  - orally: with food 0.5 g–1 g in two divided doses or 1 g daily
  - rectally: either 500 mg suppositories once daily at night or 500 mg twice daily if required
  - acute gout: initially 750 mg followed by 250 mg three times daily until the attack has subsided.
- *Children:*
  - orally: above the age of 5, 10 mg/kg daily in two divided doses
  - rectally: not recommended below 16 years of age
- *acute gout:*
  - not recommended below 16 years of age.

TIAPROFENIC ACID

Tiaprofenic acid possesses both anti-inflammatory and non-narcotic analgesic properties. It is prescribed for rheumatological disorders and other musculoskeletal conditions. Although its anti-inflammatory effects are suggested to equal those of naproxen, it is thought to have more adverse effects.

Treatment regimes

- *Adults:* orally with food 600 mg daily in 2–3 divided doses.
- *children:* not recommended

Fenamic acids

MEFENAMIC ACID

Introduced over 30 years ago Mefanamic acid is a NSAID which possesses analgesic properties. It has a half-life of 2 hours. Patients on long term therapy require haematological monitoring.

Treatment regimes

- *Adults:* orally after food 500 mg three times daily.

Salicylic acid and its derivatives

ASPIRIN

Introduced at the end of the nineteenth century, aspirin is the prototype NSAID. It is an analgesic and antipyretic and also has properties to arrest platelets forming thrombi. Currently the chief role of aspirin is as an antiplatelet drug. It is not usually prescribed as a NSAID for rheumatological conditions because of its higher prevalence of adverse effects involving the gastrointestinal tract (approximately 1 in 15 of the population) salicylism, allergy and Reye's syndrome (Laurence et al. 1997).

Treatment regimes

- *Adults:* orally with food 0.3–1 g every 4 hours with a maximum of 8 g daily for acute conditions.

BENORYLATE

Benorylate possesses anti-inflammatory, analgesic and antipyretic properties. It is derived from both aspirin and paracetamol but poses a lesser threat of gastrointestinal irritation than aspirin alone. Each 2 g of benorylate is equivalent to 920 mg of paracetamol and 1.15 g of aspirin.

Treatment regimes

Adults orally after food 4–8 g daily in 2–3 divided doses. In the elderly, total daily doses should not exceed 6 g daily.

Acetic acids

INDOMETHACIN

Introduced over 30 years ago, indomethacin has highly effective anti-inflammatory, analgesic and antipyretic properties which are considered to be superior to those of naproxen (Laurence et al. 1977).

Treatment regimes

* *Adults:*
  - orally: with food 50–200 mg daily in divided doses
  - rectally: suppositories: 100 mg twice daily
  - combined oral and rectal administration must not exceed 150–200 mg daily.
* *children:* not recommended.

DICLOFENAC

Diclofenac has anti-inflammatory and non-narcotic analgesic properties.

Treatment regime

* *Adults:*
  - orally: after food 75–150 mg daily in divided doses
  - rectally: 75–150 mg daily in divided doses
  - maximum daily dose either oral, rectal or combined should not exceed 150 mg daily.
* *Children:* below 13 years 1–3 mg/kg daily in divided doses either orally or rectally.

SULINDAC

Sulindac is both an anti-inflammatory and non-narcotic analgesic. It is a pro-drug and therefore is not highly active until it has undergone conversion in the body and gut flora. It is structurally related to indomethacin, but has fewer gastrointestinal, central nervous system and renal adverse effects (Laurence et al. 1997).

Treatment regime

* *Adults:* orally with food 200 mg twice daily, which may be reduced in relation to the clinical response. The maximum daily dose must not exceed 400 mg daily.

TOLMETIN

Tolmetin has a similar effect to ibuprofen, with anti-inflammatory, analgesic and antipyretic properties. It is recommended for pain and inflammation in rheumatic disorders, juvenile arthritis and other musculoskeletal disorders. It has a higher incidence of anaphylactic reactions than other NSAIDs, even in patients who are not allergic to aspirin or to other NSAIDs (Laurence et al. 1997).

Treatment regimes

* *Adults:* orally with food 0.6–1.8 g daily in 2–4 divided doses depending on the individual patient response and the severity of the disease. The maximum dose should not exceed 30 mg/kg daily or 1.8 g daily.
* *Children:* for juvenile arthritis, 20–25 mg/kg daily in 3–4 divided doses.

ETODOLAC

Etodolac is an anti-inflammatory and non-narcotic analgesic with a similar effect to naproxen. Its use is indicated in rheumatoid arthritis and osteoarthritis.

Treatment regimes

* *Adults:* orally with food 200–300 mg twice daily or 400–600 mg once daily. The maximum dose should not exceed 600 mg.

Enolic acids

TENOXICAM

Tenoxicam is a long-acting anti-inflammatory drug with some antipyretic properties. It is thought to inhibit prostaglandin biosynthesis and reduce leukocyte accumulation at the site of inflammation.

Treatment regime

• *Adults:* orally 20 mg once daily at the same time each day taken with water or other fluids (food reduces the rate but not the extent of absorption).
• *children:* not recommended.

PIROXICAM

Introduced nearly two decades ago, piroxicam is an anti-inflammatory and analgesic drug which is indicated for the use in rheumatic conditions and juvenile arthritis.

Treatment regime
• *Adults:*
  – orally with food 20 mg daily initially, with a maintenance dose of 10–30 mg daily either as a single or divided dose; a long-term maintenance dose of 30 mg daily increases the risk of gastrointestinal adverse effects
  – rectally: 10–20 mg daily
  – intramuscularly: recommended only on a short term basis for acute conditions
  – acute gout: 40 mg daily either as a single dose or in divided doses for 4–6 days; not recommended for the long term management of gout.
• *Children over 6 years:*
  – orally, dose depending on weight:
    below 15 kg – 5 mg daily
    16–25 kg – 10 mg daily
    26–45 kg – 15 mg daily
    over 46 kg – 20 mg daily
  – rectal and intramuscular administration not recommended.

AZAPROPAZONE

Azapropazone has anti-inflammatory, analgesic, antipyretic and uricosuric properties. However, owing to the prevalence of adverse effects, it is only recommended for rheumatoid arthritis, ankylosing spondylitis and acute gout, and only when other NSAIDs have proved not to be efficacious (Laurence et al. 1997).

Treatment regime

Adults: orally with food 1.2 g daily in 2–4 divided doses. Adults over the age of 60 or with renal impairment 300 mg twice daily.

- For acute gout, 1.8 g daily in divided doses, reducing to 1.2 g daily as the symptoms resolve. Patients with gout need to be informed that they should increase their fluid intake when they are prescribed azapropazone.
- For elderly patients and those with renal impairment, 1.8 g in divided doses for 24 hours reducing to 1.2 g daily and further reducing to a maximum dose of 600 mg daily in divided doses until the acute episode is resolved – normally by the fourth day.

Non-acidic compounds

NABUMETONE

Nabumetone is a powerful inhibitor of prostaglandin synthesis which is over 3.5 times more powerful than aspirin.

Treatment regime

- *Adults:* orally with food 1 g at night. It can be increased to 1 g twice daily in severe conditions. Elderly patients 0.5–1 g daily.

MELOXICAM

Meloxicam is a selective Cox-2 inhibitor. It is advocated for use in the short-term management of osteoarthritis and the long-term treatment of rheumatoid arthritis.

Treatment regime

- *Adults:*
  - osteoarthritis: orally with food 7.5–15 mg daily
  - rheumatoid arthritis: orally with food 7.5–15 mg daily; rectal suppositories 15 mg daily.
- *children:* not recommended under 15 years of age.

2.3 Present and future strategies in the management of rheumatoid arthritis

Use of DMARDS

A number of agents are used in attempts to control rheumatological disorders, particularly rheumatoid arthritis. Their terminology can be confusing as they are known as either *slow acting antirheumatic drugs* (SAARDs) , *second-line therapies* or *disease-modifying antirheumatic drugs* (DMARDs). In this chapter they will be referred to as DMARDs.

Despite the vast knowledge that has been amassed regarding pharmacological interventions and the disease process itself, the progression of rheumatoid arthritis remains relentless. Consequently several strategies have been developed in order to reduce the morbidity and mortality of rheumatoid arthritis. These strategies are:

- early treatment of rheumatoid arthritis with DMARDs
- combination therapy using two or more DMARDs either simultaneously or cyclically, or initial commencement of one DMARD, and if remission is not achieved, including a second DMARD in combination in order to arrest the disease process
- the use of newer/future antirheumatic agents.

Early treatment of rheumatoid arthritis

Historically, the pharmacological interventions for patients with early rheumatoid arthritis were guided by the pyramidal approach. This dictated that initial drug interventions were limited to NSAIDs and analgesics, which aimed to modify the symptoms of the disease process; hence these drugs were referred to as *symptom modifying drugs* or *first-line therapies*, and only when radiological evidence of erosions had been confirmed were DMARDs introduced into the therapeutic regime.

However, within the past decade, a consensus of opinion has challenged the traditional pyramidal approach, advocating that DMARDs should be prescribed earlier in the disease process and before rather than after any structural damage, thus minimising the disease activity quickly and effectively. The following factors suggest that the pyramidal approach should be inverted:

- There is evidence that joint destruction and concurrent functional disability occurs within the first 12 months of the disease process (Donnelley et al. 1992). Therefore it is suggested that irreversible destruction of both cartilage and bone, resulting in functional disability, rapidly occurs within the early stages of the disease process, despite the fact that rheumatoid arthritis is a chronic progressive disease. Consequently it is advocated that the optimum time to introduce DMARDs to gain control or modify the disease process is when the patient initially presents (Donnelly et al. 1992). Also, functional deterioration will occur if patients remain untreated.
- In comparison with the general population, the patient with rheumatoid arthritis has increased mortality and morbidity, which has implications not only for the individual patient (pain, disability and loss of self-esteem), but also society in general relating to loss of earnings, state payments and health care costs.

The efficacy of DMARDs in rheumatoid arthritis proves difficult to validate owing to:

- the inconsistency of the disease process
- the individual response to DMARDs
- the potential for concurrent toxic side effects.

The limited effectiveness of DMARDs may be attributed to the discontinuation of DMARD therapies because adverse effects are experienced by the patient, rather than inefficacy of the DMARDs themselves.

Combination therapy

During the last decade DMARD combination therapy has evolved owing to several factors:

- the disappointing long-term efficacy of a single DMARD regimen

- the change in philosophy entailing a more aggressive treatment regimen in an attempt to gain disease remission as early as possible.

The aim of combination therapy is to achieve a synergistic effect using two or more DMARDs in order to arrest the disease process and to achieve disease remission with minimal adverse reactions. Combination therapy can be implemented either by:

- a *step-up* regimen where one DMARD is initially prescribed and a second DMARD added if disease remission is not achieved
- a *step-down* approach entailing the initial treatment regimen of multiple DMARDs until disease suppression is achieved; the number of DMARDs can then be reduced.

Initially, combination therapy research studies targeted patients with established aggressive uncontrolled rheumatoid arthritis. However, in order to achieve maximum benefits for the maximum number of patients, research studies – although in their infancy – have been extended to include early rheumatoid arthritis patients (Haagsma et al. 1995). Table 2.6 provides examples of combination treatments in clinical practice.

Table 2.6 Combination therapies in clinical practice

Primary drug	in combination with
Gold	D-Penicillamine
	Hydroxychloroquine/chloroquine
	Methotrexate
	Azathioprine
	Sulphasalazine
	D-Penicillamine and chlorambucil
D-Penicillamine	Sulphasalazine
	Hydroxychloroquine/chloroquine
	Azathioprine
Methotrexate	Hydroxychloroquine/chloroquine
	Cyclophosphamide and chloroquine
	Azathioprine and chloroquine
Azathioprine	Sulphasalazine
	Cyclophosphamide and chloroquine

Cyclosporin has also been used in combination therapy with many agents.

Mode of action and pharmacokinetics of DMARDs

Although DMARDs can differ chemically, they have important properties in common:

- They can control the signs and symptoms of rheumatoid arthritis which include certain blood parameters denoting inflammation, painful swollen inflamed joints and sometimes slowing down the progression of radiological damage (Donnelly et al. 1992).
- Typically their action is delayed, so a therapeutic response occurs for approximately 2–4 months after treatment is started.
- All DMARDs (excluding the antimalarials) have the potential to cause serious haematological toxicity. The incidence of major or minor adverse effects consequently presents a major constraint on the continued use of these agents, so much so that approximately 20–50% of patients will have to stop their DMARD within 1 year of commencement. The safety monitoring required in the surveillance of DMARDs is discussed in depth in Chapter 3.4.

The mechanism of action of DMARD therapy is poorly understood.

The Anti-malarials

CHLOROQUINE SULPHATE/HYDROXYCHLOROQUINE SULPHATE

Chloroquine and hydroxychloroquine were originally prescribed for the treatment and prophylaxis of malaria. However, since the 1950s, research studies have revealed the efficacy of both these drugs as DMARDs in the treatment of rheumatoid arthritis and systemic lupus erythematosus (Brooks 1990). Because of their low toxicity profiles, chloroquine and hydroxychloroquine are rated as milder DMARDs which may be prescribed independently or in combination with other DMARDs when only partial efficacy is achieved. An interesting property of hydroxychloroquine, when used in combination with methotrexate, is its protective mechanism against methotrexate-induced hepatotoxicity.

Indications for use

Chloroquine and hydroxychloroquine are used in cases of:

- active rheumatoid arthritis
- juvenile arthritis
- systemic and discoid lupus erythematosus.

Treatment regime

- chloroquine: orally 250 mg daily with food
- hydroxychloroquine: orally 200–400 mg daily with food.

Retinal effect

It is generally agreed that retinal toxicity is due not to the cumulative dose, but to the daily dose. Therefore, the maximum prescription limit for adults should be 4 mg/kg per day for chloroquine and 6.5 mg/kg per day for hydroxychloroquine (Day 1994).

To prevent potential toxicity, individual physicians' regimen may differ, so patients may be prescribed chloroquine or hydroxychloroquine for 5 days of the week or for 7 days a week for 11 months of the year with a 1 month 'drug holiday'. The drug holiday will also allow the clinician to test the efficacy of the drug.

Mode of action

The mode of action of both chloroquine and hydroxychloroquine remains unknown, although research studies have suggested that antimalarials affect subcellular organelles such as polymorphs, lymphocytes and macrophages, which produce an antirheumatic and immunosuppressive reaction (Brooks 1990).

Pharmacokinetics

To avoid gastrointestinal disturbances, chloroquine and hydroxychloroquine should be administered with food. Food is not thought to affect bioavailability. Hydroxychloroquine and chloroquine accumulate extensively in tissues, and in both white and red blood cells. These medications possess above average half-lives (approximately 6 weeks), and steady concentrations are not achieved for approximately 3–4 months.

Metabolised primarily by dealkylation and thus high renal clearance, approximately 40% of chloroquine and 25% of hydroxychloroquine are excreted unchanged in the urine, therefore therapeutic regimens should be adjusted to accommodate those patients with renal impairment.

Adverse effects

The adverse effects of chloroquine and hydroxychloroquine include:

- nausea
- diarrhoea
- abdominal pain
- headaches
- dizziness
- convulsions
- blurred vision
- irreversible retinal damage
- skin reactions (rashes, pruritus)
- depigmentation or loss of hair
- ECG changes
- rarely blood disorders (thrombocytopenia, agranulocytosis, aplastic anaemia (Brooks 1990).

Contra-indications

The contra-indications of chloroquine and hydroxychloroquine include:

- psoriatic arthritis (may exacerbate psoriasis).

Monitoring

Because chloroquine and hydroxychloroquine are acknowledged as the least toxic DMARDs, the routine monitoring of blood and urine are not currently specified. Recommendations for patients on long-term therapy consist of baseline and 3–6 monthly ophthalmological examinations. Additionally, the patient could perform a monthly Amsler test. The Amsler test is a simple screening tool to detect early antimalarial induced premaculopathy, which may be reversible (Easterbrook 1988).

SULPHASALAZINE

Prescribed for patients with early rheumatoid arthritis, and in combination with other DMARDs, sulphasalazine has also been found to have some efficacy when treating seronegative spondyloarthropathies, juvenile arthritis and psoriatic arthritis (Day 1994). Developed in the 1930s when rheumatoid arthritis was thought to have an infective aetiology (Porter and Capell 1990), sulphasalazine combines an anti-inflammatory agent (5-aminosalicylic acid) and an antibiotic (sulphapyridine). However, as a result of early conflicting reports regarding the efficacy of sulphasalazine, the drug was originally dismissed by rheumatologists until the 1970s when further studies revealed its efficacy.

Mode of action

The precise mode of action of sulphasalazine is unknown, but it is thought that in some way it suppresses relevant immunological processes in the large bowel and, in addition, possesses the ability to scavenge pro-inflammatory oxygen species released from activated phagocytes (Day 1994).

Pharmacokinetics

Following oral administration the majority of the dose is absorbed in the large bowel where it reacts with colonic bacteria and separates into 5-aminosalicylic acid and sulphapyridine. Elimination is via the kidneys in the urine.

D-PENICILLAMINE

Used in the treatment of rheumatoid arthritis for 25 years, D-Penicillamine has also been useful in treating progressive systemic sclerosis as well as unrelated rheumatological conditions such as Wilson's disease, heavy metal poisoning and cystinuria.

Studies have revealed D-Penicillamine to be effective in the reduction of joint inflammation, joint pain, early morning stiffness, laboratory inflammation indices and the improvements of rheumatoid nodules (Joyce 1990).

Mode of action

For the past 25 years the precise mode of action and toxicology of D-Penicillamine has remained elusive, although it is thought to suppress the immune system (Joyce 1990).

Pharmacokinetics

D-Penicillamine is taken orally 1–2 hours before food. Peak plasma levels are present within 1–4 hours after absorption.

SODIUM AUROTHIOMALATE (GOLD)

Initially introduced and prescribed earlier this century for the treatment of tuberculosis, gold salts turned out to be of little value for that disease but were found to be efficacious for the treatment of rheumatoid arthritis. Sodium Aurothiomalate has been shown to impede progressive radiological damage and concomitant functional impairment in both short and medium term treatment of rheumatoid arthritis, although its efficacy in long term treatment is questionable (Day 1994).

Mode of action

To date there is no consensus on the precise mode of action of intramuscular gold, although it is known to regulate gene transcription and affect polymorphonuclear and synovial cells, monocytes, lymphocytes and immunoglobins (Champion et al. 1990, Day 1994).

Pharmacokinetics

Gold is polymeric and therefore not absorbed orally. Following intramuscular injection absorption takes place quickly and gold travels to synovial tissue where it binds to inflamed synovial tissues; consequently, most of the gold is located in the synovial lining cells. Elimination is initially rapid and largely in the urine. However, gold has been detected in tissues some 20 years after therapy.

AURANOFIN

Auranofin is a gold-based drug that can be taken orally. Although considered less efficacious than sodium aurothiomalate, D-Penicillamine or methotrexate, auranofin has fewer serious side effects. (Champion et al. 1990).

Mode of action

As with sodium aurothiomalate, the precise mode of action remains elusive.

Pharmacokinetics

Following oral administration of auranofin, absorption is rapid but incomplete; only 20–25% of the gold is absorbed (Blocka et al. 1982). Approximately 15% is then excreted via the kidneys, but most of the gold is excreted in the faeces which contain both unabsorbed drug and gold that has been absorbed in the gastrointestinal tract and bound to gastric epithelium (Champion et al. 1990, Day 1994).

METHOTREXATE

Initially introduced some 50 years ago for the treatment of acute leukaemia, methotrexate is classed as one of the first antimetabolites. It was introduced as a treatment for rheumatoid arthritis in the 1950s; however, it was not until the 1980s that methotrexate was used widely by rheumatologists for the treatment of rheumatoid arthritis and psoriatic arthritis.

Mode of action

Methotrexate is a cytotoxic drug which acts as a folate antagonist to cause cell death by affecting the synthesis of DNA. However, its precise mode of action in the treatment of rheumatoid arthritis is not entirely understood.

Pharmacokinetics

Following administration (oral or intramuscular), methotrexate is absorbed rapidly and almost entirely, taking 1–2 hours before a peak concentration is achieved. Most excretion is via the kidneys, but biliary elimination is suggested to account for approximately 10–30% of the methotrexate (Songsiridej and Furst 1990).

AZATHIOPRINE

Azathioprine is a cytotoxic immunosuppressant drug, originally prescribed to prevent the rejection of transplanted organs. It has also proved to be efficacious in the treatment of rheumatoid arthritis, vasculitis, systemic lupus erythematosus, polymyalgia rheumatica/ giant cell arteritis, Behçet's disease, polymyositis, dermatomyositis, myasthenia gravis and chronic inflammatory bowel disease.

Mode of action

The precise mode of action of azathioprine is unclear but, as an immunosuppressant, it interferes with DNA synthesis either by inhibiting cell division or by causing cell death in relation to rheumatoid arthritis. This results in fewer circulating B and T lymphocytes (Furst and Clements 1994, Luqmani et al. 1990). Azathioprine is also administered as a steroid-sparing agent.

Pharmacokinetics

Following oral administration, azathioprine remains inactive until it is metabolised in the liver into 6-thioinosinic acid and 6-thioguanylic acid. Elimination is via the kidneys.

CYCLOPHOSPHAMIDE

Cyclophosphamide, a derivative of nitrogen mustard, is an alkylating agent which was developed in the 1940s as an anticancer drug.

It has been shown to possess both immunosuppressive and immunostimulatory effects (Miller and North 1981, Turk and Parker 1979). Its use by rheumatologists for the treatment of rheumatoid arthritis began in the late 1960s, even though research studies revealed conflicting results regarding its efficacy in controlling or slowing down radiographic changes. Cyclophosphamide has proved to be effective in the treatment of the systemic complications of rheumatoid arthritis, such as vasculitis, and it has also proved to be effective in the treatment of systemic lupus erythematosus (Austin et al. 1986).

Mode of action

The mode of action of cyclophosphamide is not entirely understood; it is known to crosslink DNA and act to stop DNA replication and halt cell division. Additionally, it has a toxic effect on resting cells. This is said to account for its quick action which is accompanied by greater toxicity than azathioprine (Brookes 1990, Furst and Clements 1994).

Pharmacokinetics

Cyclophosphamide may be administered orally or intravenously. It is predominantly metabolised in the liver, and to some extent also in the kidneys and lungs (Bagley et al. 1973). It is excreted via the faeces, expiration, spinal fluid, perspiration, breast milk, saliva and synovial fluid (Furst and Clements 1994). Most, however, is excreted by the kidneys either unchanged (less than 20%) or as metabolites in the urine (65%). The dominant metabolite of cyclophosphamide (acrolein) has been highlighted as the major source of bladder toxicity (Mouridsen and Jacobsen 1975) and hence an increased fluid intake is essential when this drug is administered.

CYCLOSPORIN

Cyclosporin is an immunosuppressant, initially developed to suppress the rejection of organ transplantation. Its antiarthritis properties were initially identified in the mid-1970s (Borel et al. 1976). Further studies have demonstrated that it can reduce bone and cartilage destruction (Del Pozo et al. 1990) and also restore T-helper and T-suppressor subsets (Bersani-Amado et al. 1990, Yocum et al. 1986). Cyclosporin has been used in the treatment of rheumatoid arthritis and retinal vasculitis, including that witnessed in Behcet's syndrome.

Mode of action

Cyclosporin can inhibit T-cell response and interaction by blocking interleukin-2 and other pro-inflammatory cytokines.

Pharmacokinetics

When cyclosporin is taken orally, absorption is both incomplete and erratic (Kowal et al. 1990) with distribution taking place outside rather than inside the blood volume; hence, it has been detected in the body fat, liver, lungs, kidneys, adrenal glands, spleen and lymph nodes. Consequently elimination is mainly via the biliary system and, to a much lesser extent, via the urine (Furst and Clements 1994).

CHLORAMBUCIL

Although generally out of vogue in the UK for the past 20 years, chlorambucil has maintained its popularity in France and North America for the treatment of most connective tissue disease and associated inflammatory eye diseases (Luqmani et al. 1990).

Mode of action

Chlorambucil is a cytotoxic drug (a nitrogen mustard derivative) and belongs to the group of drugs known as alkylating agents. Alkylating agents are chemically very active substances which bind with DNA within the cell nucleus resulting in cell death at the point of cell division.

Pharmacokinetics

Administered orally, chlorambucil is rapidly absorbed; both unchanged chlorambucil and its metabolites are excreted in the urine.

PHENYLBUTAZONE

Introduced in 1949 for the treatment of arthritis and gout, phenylbutazone is said to be one of the oldest and strongest NSAIDs and is often prescribed for its suppressive properties. However, because of reported toxic side effects, it is currently only prescribed for ankylosing spondylitis under hospital specialist supervision.

Mode of action

Phenlbutazone acts to inhibit the biosynthesis of prostaglandins (Moll 1983).

Pharmacokinetics

Administered orally with food (because of gastric irritation), like other NSAIDs, phenylbutazone is almost entirely absorbed from the gastrointestinal tract (as it is not bound irretrievably by food). Elimination is via the kidneys following conversion by the liver (Hart and Klinenberg 1985).

DAPSONE

Known principally as an antileprotic drug, dapsone has also proved effective as an antimalarial, and in the treatment of both rheumatoid arthritis and psoriatic arthritis.

Mode of action

Related to sulphonamide antibacterials, dapsone produces a depressant effect on the immune system.

Pharmacokinetics

Taken orally, dapsone is absorbed rapidly, with excretion via the kidneys in the urine.

MINOCYCLINE

Minocycline is a broad spectrum antibiotic, prescribed for the treatment of tetracycline-sensitive organisms, certain strains of meningitis, acne and rheumatoid arthritis.

Mode of action

The mode of action of minocycline is unclear but it is thought to inhibit pro-inflammatory enzymes.

Pharmacokinetics

Following absorption, minocycline spreads widely throughout the body, including a variable penetration across the meningeal barrier into the cerebrospinal fluid. Excretion of most of the drug is slowly via the kidneys.

Newer/future treatments of rheumatoid arthritis

In an attempt to produce more effective antirheumatic treatments, a number of different strategies are currently being adapted. They include:

- new immunosuppressive drugs
- monoclonal antibodies
- chemical cytokine modifiers
- arachidonic acid metabolite modifiers
- oral tolerance.

New immunosuppressive drugs

A number of new immunosuppressive drugs are currently being developed or evaluated in clinical trials. These include:

- Leflunomide, a drug which possesses various immunomodulatory effects that seem related to the inhibition of lymphokine signal transduction
- FK506, another new immunosuppressive drug which possesses cyclosporin-like properties and is currently being evaluated within the field of transplant surgery and, like cyclosporin, may also prove of value for patients with rheumatological disorders.

Monoclonal antibodies

Much interest has been generated in the role of T lymphocytes in rheumatoid arthritis, because research has suggested that T lymphocytes or their products initiate the inflammatory process. Consequently studies have been conducted to deplete T cells by various methods (Karsh et al. 1981, Nusslein et al. 1985, Paulus et al. 1977, Wilder and Decker 1983). All studies reported a significant clinical improvement following the depletion of T cells. This knowledge has led to the development of agents that target surface antigens, in particular specific monoclonal antibodies (MAb) which are specific for certain cell surface markers such as CD4 which are expressed by T-helper cells. Research studies involving CD4-MAb have demonstrated some success with an immediate and prolonged reduction in the amount of circulating T cells, which was mirrored by an immediate and prolonged reduction in disease activity.

Other specific MAb therapy is anti-TNF which is specific for the pro-inflammatory cytokine tumour necrosis factor (TNF). Studies involving intravenous infusion of TNF demonstrated promising results, with 60% of subjects experiencing improvements in measurements of inflammation and function and an almost immediate reduction of both pain and tiredness (Elliot et al. 1994).

Following the promising results of specific MAb, it appears quite possible that in the future a variety or a 'cocktail' of MAbs, each controlling a different aspect of the immune response, will be advocated in the management of rheumatoid arthritis. However, this will only be possible after long-term studies to demonstrate both the long term efficacy and safety of specific MAb therapy (Breedveld 1997).

Chemical cytokine modifiers

Pro-inflammatory cytokines (e.g. TNF, interleukin-1) have been identified which appear to possess a central role in the pathology of rheumatoid arthritis; this has led to research into the development of therapeutic potential inhibitors of these cytokines. Certain cytokines (e.g. interleukin-10) have been shown to exert an important immunoregulatory effect, hence research regarding the therapeutic inhibitors of these specific cytokines are taking place, although currently in their infancy (Breeddveld 1997).

Arachidonic acid metabolite modifiers

Within the field of prostaglandin inhibition, one development has been the advent of specific COX-2 inhibitors to minimise toxicity (by not inhibiting COX-1) while retaining efficacy. Additionally, agents such as Tenidap have been developed that not only inhibit Cox-2 but also inhibit certain pro-inflammatory cytokines. In clinical trials Tenidap has been shown to improve the signs and symptoms of active rheumatoid arthritis within one month of treatment by decreasing pain and stiffness, the number of active joints and inflammatory markers such as the erythrocyte sedimentation rate (ESR).

Oral tolerance

The concept of immunological tolerance is currently being explored in rheumatoid arthritis therapeutic studies. Immunological tolerance represents the ability of the body's immune system to fail to react to a specific molecule which would normally be antigenic. For example, in animal studies guinea pigs normally respond to the injection of foreign (dietary) protein with an allergic reaction. However, prior feeding of high doses of the protein prevents this allergic reaction on subsequent injection of the protein. This tolerance is specific for that protein, other foreign proteins would evoke an allergic response.

Within the realms of rheumatology the concept of oral tolerance would be to build up a tolerance to the target antigens at which the autoimmune response is directed. One possible target in rheumatoid arthritis would be articular cartilage, and studies are currently taking place using Type II chicken collagen as the agent for increasing tolerance.

Summary

Research involving the pathophysiology of rheumatoid arthritis has enabled many exciting therapeutic developments which aim to provide better control of both the disease symptoms and the disease progression. Currently, however, although this is certainly true in the short and medium term, longer-term control of the disease process or a cure for rheumatoid arthritis remain elusive.

2.4 Use of steroids in the treatment of rheumatic disease

Corticosteroid drugs are synthetic derivatives of the body's naturally occurring corticosteroid hormones which are produced in the cortex of the adrenal glands. The principal corticosteroid of the human adrenal cortex is *cortisol* (*hydrocortisone*), derived from the hydroxylation of cortisone. The adrenal gland production of corticosteroids is controlled by the hypothalamus and the pituitary gland via a negative feedback system. Corticosteroids comprise androgenic steroids, mineralocorticoids and glucocorticoids.

Glucocorticoids

The glucocorticoids are responsible for:

- carbohydrate, protein and fat metabolism
- maintenance of blood sugar levels
- the body's response to both physical and psychological stress
- suppression of inflammation and the immune response (Christiansen and Krane 1993).

The properties and the synthetic manufacture of glucocorticoids for the treatment of rheumatoid arthritis has been of interest to rheumatologists for the last six decades. Much research has taken place to isolate the glucocorticoid that possesses precise anti-inflammatory and immunosuppressive properties, but to date it remains elusive.

The role of systemic steroids in the management of rheumatological disorders is complex because, although they are very effective anti-inflammatory and immunosuppressive agents, even with relatively low doses they are also associated with potentially serious side effects which may cause significant morbidity.

Systemic steroids currently prescribed in the treatment of rheumatological disorders include *hydrocortisone (cortisol), prednisolone, cortisone* and *methyl prednisolone.*

Mode of action

Corticosteroids act by binding to specific cytoplasmic receptors which then enter the nucleus where they cause the production of certain mRNAs coding for various proteins. The beneficial effects of systemic steroids are partly related to increased production of lipocortin and decreased production of the inflammatory response, e.g. cytokines, prostaglandins and leukotrienes (see Figure 2.3).The exact effects on the lymphocyte function are still poorly understood. It is not yet possible to separate different corticosteroid effects by using different corticosteroid analogues, indicating that their actions are similar and their relative potencies relate to their structure and plasma half-life (Kirwan 1994) – see Table 2.7.

Corticosteroid-sparing agents

Drugs which are prescribed in order to make it easier to reduce the corticosteroid dose, while at the same time controlling the underlying disease, are known as corticosteroid-sparing agents (Kirwan et al. 1995). Azathioprine, cyclophosphamide and methotrexate can all be used for this purpose.

Adverse effects of corticosteroids

Immune system

Corticosteroids are powerful immunosuppressants which affect both humoral and cell mediated immune responses. Although corticosteroids can be valuable in the treatment of autoimmune diseases they can also be potentially life threatening because high levels of

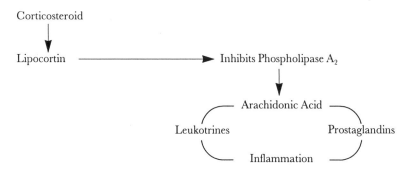

Figure 2.3 The action of corticosteroids.

Table 2.7 Half life of commonly used corticosteroids

Corticosteroids	half life (hours)
Short acting Cortisone Cortisol	8–12

Intermediate acting
Prednisolone
    Prednisone
    Methylprednisolone
    Triamcinolone
	12–36

Long acting
Paramethasone
    Dexamethasone
    Betamethasone
	36–72

corticosteroids will also reduce the formation of antibodies and the white cell production of patients, thus permitting the invasion of bacteria or viruses and the spread of infection. Patients on long-term corticosteroids may also be predisposed to staphylococcal, gram-negative, tuberculous and listeria infections (Christiansen and Krane 1993, Kirwan 1994) (see Table 2.8)

Glucose metabolism

The problem of glucose intolerance with patients receiving corticosteroids was initially highlighted in the late 1940s. The suggested mechanisms of glucose intolerance are:

- decreased insulin secretion
- increased hepatic glucose production
- impaired peripheral glucose metabolism.

Bone mineral metabolism

Studies have revealed that cytoplasmic glucocorticoid receptors are present in bone cells which appear to influence calcium intake and excretion and the factors that regulate hormones, cytokines and growth factors. Therefore, prolonged steroid therapy possesses multifaceted adverse effects on bone mineral metabolism which precipitate growth retardation in children, osteoporosis, long bone and vertebral fractures. The adverse effects of steroids that affect bone material metabolism include their effects on:

Table 2.8 Adverse effects of corticosteroids

System	Side effect	Comment
Metabolic	Obesity	Changes due to fat redistribution result in cushingoid features such as moon face
	Glucose/protein metabolism	Hyperglycaemia and insulin resistance occur
Decreased resistance to infection		Due to immunosuppression. Candida and herpes zoster infection has occurred in patients taking corticosteroids, along with a variety of bacterial infections
Musculoskeletal	Muscle wastage	Due to protein catabolism
	Tendon rupture	Occurs with direct injection into tendon
	Osteoporosis	Due to a reduction in calcium absorption into the bones and increase in calcium excretion. Vertebral wedge and crush fractures are a frequent complication of treatment
	Corticosteroid withdrawal syndrome	Occurs with long term use of steroids (more than 7 days) and as a result of too rapid withdrawal. Symptoms include myalgia, fatigue, malaise, anorexia, nausea, weight loss. Recommend a slow withdrawal appropriate to the length of time a patient has been on the steroid
Gastrointestinal	Peptic ulceration	Due to the inhibition of gastric prostaglandins which maintain the integrity of the gastric mucosa
	Pancreatitis	
Ophthalmic	Cataracts	
	Glaucoma	
Central nervous system	Psychosis	A paranoid and suicidal state may be induced by steroids
	Euphoria	
	Depression	
Skin	Acne	
	Striae	Due to protein catabolism. A symptom of cushingoid side effects.
	Alopecia	
	Bruising	
	Skin atrophy	Due to protein catabolism
Growth retardation		
Adrenal suppression		

- *Osteoblasts:* Steroid therapy has been shown to reduce circulating osteocalcin levels which affect osteoblast activity thus inhibiting bone formation. Studies have also revealed that bone matrix synthesis is affected within 24 hours of the administration of steroids (Reid et al. 1986, Godschalk and Downs 1988).
- *Osteoclasts:* Steroid therapy is thought to have a dual accelerating effect on bone reabsorption either by directly stimulating osteoclasts or indirectly under the influence of parathyroid hormone (PTH).
- *Gastrointestinal absorption of calcium:* The consensus of opinion is that steroids suppress the intestinal absorption of calcium although the reason remains unclear.
- *Excretion of calcium:* A decrease in the reabsorption of calcium within the kidneys has been shown to occur in patients. Although glucocorticoid receptors are present in the kidney, their precise mode of action on calcium reabsorption/excretion is unclear (Fuller and Funder 1976).
- *Vitamin D:* Extensive research regarding the effects of steroids and 25-hydroxyvitamin D levels have revealed conflicting evidence, hence the suggested osteopenic effects of steroids in relation to 25-hydroxyvitamin D levels remains controversial.
- *Parathyroid hormone:* Parathyroid hormone regulates blood phosphorus and calcium levels via its actions on the intestines, bone tissue and kidneys. A normal concentration of calcium (2.2–2.6 mmol/l) is essential for normal physiology. However, numerous studies have demonstrated that steroids stimulate the parathyroid glands and increase parathyroid hormone levels, which stimulates osteoclasts to accelerate bone resorption (Cosman et al. 1992).
- *Growth retardation:* Since the early 1950s growth retardation in children has been a recognised side effect of long term steroid therapy, although the precise mechanisms remain elusive. It is suggested that steroid therapy has a direct effect, and an indirect consequence on both the osteoblast and cartilage cells which consequently suppresses the growth of linear bone and impedes epiphyseal closure (Loeb 1976). The prevention of growth retardation is helped by prescribing an alternate day regimen (Polito et al. 1986, Guest and Broyer 1991).
- *Bone loss:* Studies in adults treated with corticosteroids do not clearly suggest a threshhold dose below which osteoporosis can be avoided (Kirwan 1994), although there does appear to be a consistent relationship between doses above 7.5 mg daily and the rate of bone loss.

Peptic ulceration

Evidence from controlled studies of corticosteroid therapy suggests that the increased risk of peptic ulceration is considerably lower than is widely believed (Cooper and Kirwan 1990). However, corticosteroids may exacerbate the ulcergenic properties of NSAIDs (Piper et al. 1991).

Atherosclerosis

Prolonged corticosteroid therapy may accelerate the development of atherosclerosis (Cooper and Kirwan 1990), with lower limb atherosclerosis occurring in as many as 60% of corticosteroid treated patients with rheumatoid arthritis. The evidence linking corticosteroid therapy with atherosclerosis is still considered controversial but, in time, even a small effect could have considerable clinical significance.

Methods of administration

A number of administration routes are available for corticosteroids:

- oral
- intravenous pulses
- intramuscular injections
- intra-articular injections
- soft tissue injections.

Intravenous pulses

Pulse therapy involves the intravenous infusion of a large dose of corticosteroid (usually 500 mg–1 g of methylprednisolone) over 30–60 minutes. There are many different treatment regimens in practice but most include a course of three pulses on alternate days, followed by a resting phase of around 6 weeks (Kirwan et al. 1995). It may be used to bridge the time interval between initiation and response to DMARDs or, when patients have an acute flare of their rheumatoid arthritis, to induce remission. A review of the use of pulsed methylprednisolone (Weusten et al. 1993) shows few or minor side effects. Those who have experienced severe adverse effects of the cardiovascular system, or experienced infection, had existing compromised cardiovascular and immune systems as a result of their disease or due to concomitant drug therapy (Kirwan et al. 1995).

Intramuscular injections

Intramuscular injections of corticosteroid may be used to reduce the symptoms of a flare in rheumatoid arthritis, or administered prior to the initiation of DMARD therapy where it is known that these medications take many months before benefit can be assessed. It is important to give the injection deep into the muscle to prevent muscular atrophy occurring. Choy et al. (1993) found that intramuscular methylprednisolone was superior to equivalent oral doses in their study of corticosteroids and gold therapy.

Intra-articular injections

Intra-articular and soft tissue injections are interventions used in the management of rheumatology disorders. In comparison to oral corticosteroids, they are well tolerated and safe if administered appropriately. The Royal College of Nursing Rheumatology Forum has produced guidelines on the use and administration of intra-articular injections, (see appendix, pp. 138–40).

Treatment regimen

The factors that dictate the treatment regimen for corticosteroids include the actual disease, its severity and the clinical response. Kirwan (1994) divides the treatment regime into three dose-related ranges:

- low daily doses (up to 15 mg) to treat polymyalgia and symptomatic rheumatoid arthritis
- high daily doses (20–60 mg) for serious disease, e.g. temporal arteritis, dermatomyositis, lupus erythematosus
- very high doses (pulsed methylprednisolone) for acute or life-threatening crisis.

Reducing the dose of corticosteroids

High doses of corticosteroids are often used for only short periods and can be reduced rapidly with little adverse effect. The exact mode of reduction will depend on the control of the clinical situation. Patients treated with moderate to low doses of corticosteroid over a longer duration of time may develop a corticosteroid withdrawal syndrome when their treatment is reduced. This can include the symptoms of myalgia, fatigue and nausea and has been reported in as many as 70% of patients treated with 30 mg prednisolone daily for longer than 3 months. (Dixon and Christy 1980).

One approach to try and avoid this is to reduce the corticosteroid treatment very slowly, often by as little as 2.5 mg daily every 2 months down to 7.5 mg daily, then introduce further graduated reductions of 1 mg daily or on alternate days.

The administration of exogenous steroids may result in the suppression of the body's own (endogenous) steroid production. Therefore, when exogenous steroids are withdrawn, the adrenal gland may fail to produce adequate cortisol, resulting in a steroid crisis with a failure of cortisol production. This in turn results in hypotension, hypoglycaemia and electrolyte imbalance. All patients on steroid treatment should carry a steroid card with them.

The withdrawal of steroids can lead to a marked flare in symptoms of the disease process which may necessitate the patient being recommenced on steroids.

Pharmacokinetics

Following oral administration of prednisolone, absorption takes place quickly within the gastrointestinal tract and is rapidly metabolised within the liver, with excretion via the urine. Its action on the tissues is of a much longer duration than its presence in the blood (George and Kirwan 1990).

Drug interactions

- *NSAIDs:* risk of gastrointestinal irritation increased
- *Antibacterials:* reduce the effect of corticosteroids
- *Antidiabetic drugs:* effect inhibited
- *Antiepileptics:* reduce the effect of corticosteroids
- *Antihypertensives:* effect inhibited
- *Cyclosporin:* increased plasma concentration of prednisolone and cyclosporin
- *Diuretics:* effect inhibited
- *Anticoagulants:* effect may be enhanced or reduced
- *Vaccines:* live vaccines should not be administered to patients receiving corticosteroids.

Corticosteroids in the management of rheumatic disease

Rheumatoid arthritis

Corticosteroids are the only medications which reliably, effectively and rapidly reduce synovitis in rheumatoid arthritis (Kirwan et al. 1995). In a review of clinical trials of corticosteroids in rheumatoid arthritis it was concluded that in both short- and long-term studies corticosteroids are effective inflammatory agents, significantly better than placebo and NSAIDs in the relief of pain and stiffness (George and Kirwan 1990). However, the problem with using steroids for control of synovitis is that benefits are not sustained unless increasing doses are employed. This increases the risk of steroid side effects and it often becomes very difficult to decrease or stop the steroids.

Kirwan et al. (1995) demonstrated that patients with early rheumatoid arthritis who received prednisolone 7.5 mg daily experienced less radiological joint damage (in the hands) than did those individuals receiving placebo. This study has reopened the debate on the use of steroids in the management of rheumatoid arthritis.

Polymyalgia rheumatica and temporal arteritis

The symptoms of polymyalgia rheumatica and temporal arteritis often overlap. No controlled trials have been conducted to provide guidance on the best treatment dosage with corticosteroids (Kirwan 1994). Although practice will differ, polymyalgia rheumatica is often treated with an initial dose of 15 mg prednisolone daily reducing slowly over 18–24 months governed by blood inflammatory parameters and clinical symptoms. One potential problem is to commence too high a dose of prednisolone accompanied by too rapid a reduction in dosage over time. This will often result in an exacerbation of original symptoms.

The treatment of temporal arteritis requires a much higher dose of steroid, usually 60–100 mg daily.

Collagenosis

The use of steroids is largely determined by the nature of the collagenosis complication rather than by the collagenosis itself – e.g. in the case of systemic lupus erythematosus many individuals with mild disease manifestations may not require steroids.

Inflammatory muscle diseases

Dermatomysitis and polymyositis patients are treated with medium to high daily dose steroids initially. This will often be accompanied with a cytotoxic agent such as azathioprine or methotrexate.

Vasculitis

Management of vasculitis involving major organs (e.g. Wegner's granulomatosis, rheumatoid vasculitis, polyarteritis nodosa) will necessitate the use of high dose steroids orally or as a intravenous pulse therapy to induce remission.

2.5 Gout

Gout is a metabolic disorder in which an acute monarthritic condition occurs when the blood plasma contains increased levels of uric acid (*hyperuricaemia*). Uric acid is the product of purine metabolism, and hyperuricaemia can occur either from an overproduction of uric acid (20–25% of patients) or when the kidneys fail to excrete uric acid (75% of patients). Excessive hyperuricaemia may then result in the formation of uric acid crystals which are deposited in various parts of the body: most commonly in the joints of the foot, hand and knee, although the crystals may also form tophi in soft tissues or stones in the kidney (Edwards and Boucher 1991).

Epidemiology

In Britain the prevalence of gout is approximately 0.1%, with males outnumbering females by 8 : 1. The mean age of onset is 40 for men and 70 for women. The majority of men experience primary gout (no obvious cause) whereas women tend to experience secondary gout (e.g. diuretic induced).

Clinical features

About 70% of patients present with an acute attack of gout, which is typically characterised by a sudden onset of *podagra* (an acute, red, painful swelling at the metatarsophalangeal joint of the great toe), although the knees and hands may also be affected. Patients with acute attacks may also present with a raised erythrocyte sedimentation rate (ESR), pyrexia and leucocytosis.

Precipitating factors

There are many precipitating factor for an attack of gout, including:

- a raised level of uric acid (greater than 430 over 10 mg/dl mol/l), resulting either from an oversecretion from the liver or impaired kidney excretion
- obesity
- alcohol
- hypertension
- severe dietary restriction
- diuretics
- a sudden fall of uric acid levels following the administration of allopurinol or uricosuric drugs
- trauma
- surgery
- severe systemic illness.

Chronic gout

If episodes of acute gout reoccur and remain untreated, gout develops into a chronic condition in which erosions of both cartilage and bone may occur along with deposits of tophi. Tophi are composed of sodium biurate and appear as small hard chalky or cheesy deposits which may discharge and ulcerate. Consequently, chronic gout may result in joint deformities and subsequent functional impairment.

Diagnosis

The examination of synovial fluid by polarised light microscopy is used to identify monosodium uric acid crystals. The identification of these crystals provides the clinician with a definite diagnosis of gout, thus excluding either sepsis or *pseudogout*. The crystals present in pseudogout are calcium pyrophosphate. The correct diagnosis is paramount to ensure that patients are not prescribed treatment unnecessarily (Currey 1988).

Diagnostic features of gout include hyperuricaemia (although not all patients with hyperuricaemia have gout).

Radiographs in early acute attacks are unremarkable. However, the appearance of classic 'punched out' erosions (radiolucent urate tophi) appears later with chronic gout.

Following subsequent episodes of gout, examination of the patient may reveal tophaceous deposits in the helix of the ear, bursae, tendon sheaths and kidney parenchyma.

Treatment

The management of gout is planned in two stages; initially the management of the acute inflammatory joint symptoms, and secondly the long-term management of persistent hyperuricaemia.

First-stage treatment

The aim of initial therapy is to suppress the inflammatory process induced by the deposit of uric acid crystals which may be present in and around joints, in tendons and in the kidney parenchyma. Hence, NSAIDs are the first line of treatment. The NSAID prescribed will depend on both the patient's tolerance, and the clinician's preference and, although many NSAIDs have been found to be equally efficacious, indomethacin is generally accepted as the NSAID of choice in the treatment of acute gout (Gibson 1988). Following commencement of NSAID therapy, pain begins to subside within 2 hours, and control of the inflammation is gained within 2–14 days (mode of action, side effects and contraindications of NSAIDs are discussed in the Chapter 2.2).

COLCHICINE

If NSAIDs are contra-indicated, colchicine is prescribed. Derived from the autumn crocus *Colchicum autumnale*, this is an ancient remedy which has been prescribed since the eighteenth century for the treatment of gout (Emmerson 1994).

Mode of action

Colchicine is an alkaloid which halts both the inflammatory response and the deposit of uric acid crystals, although its precise mode of action is complicated and not entirely understood.

Pharmacokinetics

Following administration, colchicine is absorbed through the upper small bowel, metabolised by the liver and then excreted both in the bile and intestinal secretions. As 20% is excreted unchanged in the urine, the dose of colchicine should be adjusted accordingly for those patients who have pre-existing renal disease (Emmerson 1994).

Treatment regimen

Initially patients are prescribed 1 mg, followed by 0.5 mg every 2 hours, which usually has an effect within 24 hours of commencement of therapy. However, because the therapeutic regimen may mirror the toxic dose, dosage continues until either:

- the maximum total dose is attained (10 mg)
- the gout subsides
- side effects are experienced (diarrhoea and vomiting).

NB: Colchicine 0.5 mg 2–3 times daily may also be prescribed concurrent with initial long term treatment of hypouricaemic drugs to prevent further attack of acute gout. Adverse effects are shown in Table 2.9.

Drug interactions

- *Cyclosporin:* increased plasma levels – therefore possible risk of both nephrotocixity and myotoxicity.

Second-stage therapy: long-term treatment

The aim of long term treatment of gout is to prevent the possible consequences of further episodes of acute gout (joint deformity, loss of joint function, and kidney damage).

The hypouricaemic drug most commonly prescribed is allopurinol which is a xanthine oxidase inhibitor which acts to inhibit the production of uric acid. Other hypouricaemic drugs include probenecid and sulphinpyrazone, which are both uricosuric drugs that block the tubular reabsorption of filtered urate in the kidneys and therefore increase the excretion of uric acid via the kidneys. Second-stage therapy, therefore, is prescribed to prevent reoccurring

Table 2.9 Adverse effects of colchicine

Nausea/vomiting
Abdominal pain
Gastrointestinal haemorrhage
Rashes
Renal and hepatic impairment
Peripheral neuritis
Myopathy
Blood disorders(with prolonged therapy)

acute attacks of gout by maintaining uric acid levels that fall within normal blood plasma parameters.

Indications for the prescription of second-stage therapy are:

- hyperuricaemia with recurrent episodes of acute gout
- visible tophi and/or erosions revealed by radiological examination
- associated renal impairment.

ALLOPURINOL

Allopurinol acts by inhibiting xanthine oxidase, the product that enables the conversion of xanthine and hypoxanthine to uric acid (Edwards and Boucher 1991). Because of its low incidence of side effects, allopurinol is the most widely used drug for the long-term prophylaxis of gout. Its added advantage is that it can also be prescribed for those patients with renal impairment or those who have kidney stones.

Treatment regimen

The dose of allopurinol is 100 mg once daily, initially for one week (initial dose for both the elderly and patients with renal dysfunction should be reduced to 50 mg to prevent toxicity, Gibson 1988), increasing over 2–3 weeks to a maintenance dose (dependent on either blood plasma or urinary uric levels) of 200–600 mg daily in divided doses. Tablets should be taken after food.

Uricosuric drugs

PROBENCID

Treatment regimen
- week 1: 250 mg twice daily
- week 2: 500 mg twice daily.

Maintenance dose up to 2 g daily in divided doses according to uric acid levels. Tablets are to be taken after food.

SULPHINPYRAZONE

Treatment regimen

Initially 100–200 mg daily, increasing over 2–3 weeks to 600 mg daily.

It may be possible to reduce the maintenance dose (when uric acid blood plasma falls within normal levels) to 200 mg daily. Tablets to be taken with either food or milk.

Compliance

Compliance with long-term therapy is dependent on patient education regarding the differing actions of both initial and long-term therapies. To prevent further attacks of gout, patients should receive health promotion regarding the risk factors that can precipitate an acute episode of gout.

2.6 Self-medication and complementary medicine

Self-medication

If the treatment of rheumatoid arthritis is to be effective, patients must have the ability to adjust drug administration according to the changing activity of their disease (Hill et al. 1991). Awareness and knowledge of prescribed medications is important in aiding compliance. It is vital in patients with chronic inflammatory conditions who take medications for a long period of time, as there is a clear need to assess both the safety and the efficacy of the drug regime (Hopkins 1990), especially as it is the patient who will be responsible for administering prescribed medications at home. Healthcare professionals can no longer assume that people are passive recipients of care, and patients will require information to administer medicines safely and effectively (Kennedy 1981).

Beardsley et al. (1983) define drug self-administration procedures as specific education strategies that contain the necessary knowledge and behavioural components to effect better compliance. (The whole area of compliance is discussed in further depth in Chapter 4.)

The case for self-medication

The conventional system of drug administration from a ward trolley often neglects to address the need for individual education, nor does it seek to prepare patients to administer drugs within their own home environment following discharge. All the nurse has to do is to administer and sign that the prescribed drug has been given. This is despite the fact that health education has become a major part of the nurse's role (Bird 1990). This traditional system frequently provides dosages at incorrect times, and unfortunately is not error free (Johnson and Giles 1993). It should no longer be acceptable to the profession and we should aim to provide patients with a personal pharmacy

(Corrigan 1989). Webb (1990) states that the traditional approach of batch processing suits staff convenience rather than being governed by patient need, whereas a holistic humanitarian approach to nursing care necessitates considering people as individuals and providing care in partnership with them.

An important but often neglected area of discharge planning is whether a patient is being discharged home without adequate knowledge of their tablets or, quite possibly, with containers that they cannot open. The United Kingdom Central Council has recommended that self-administration projects be established during a hospital stay to provide patients with the necessary knowledge and confidence to continue with a high degree of compliance on discharge (Sutherland et al. 1991).

A large number of patients fail to adhere to drug regimens (Evans and Spelman 1983, Eraker et al. 1984) with the consequence that, in more than a third of cases, the patient's health is actually endangered (Stewart and Cliff 1977). Parkin et al. (1976) studied 130 patients following discharge, 66 of whom deviated from their prescribed regime. In 46 of these cases it was because the patients did not understand the instructions on how to take their tablets.

Many patients, particularly older people, are taking medications when they are admitted to hospital. Unfortunately, 25–59% of these patients will be making errors in their drug administration (Stewart and Cliff 1977). Hopkins (1990) also found that patients' knowledge (of those attending a rheumatology outpatient clinic) decreased with age and 35% of patients aged over 75 had no knowledge at all about their medication. Many of these patients were taking NSAIDs which require knowledge for safe management.

Quilligan (1990) offers a framework for ensuring that the older patient is given enough support in learning about their tablets. It follows the structure of the nursing process:

Patient assessment

• Does the patient understand his or her condition and the purpose of the medications?
• Does the patient want to learn more about his or her medications and can he or she do so?
• Can the family be involved in the process?

Planning and implementation

- Use realistic joint goals on agreed topics and if possible conduct the sessions when the family can be present.
- Limit the teaching to 3 topics in a 15 minute maximum session.
- Discuss the patient's worries and check previous knowledge.

Evaluation

- Ongoing assessment of managing tablets and the teaching programme is required.

Advantages of self-medication

Patients have the chance to familiarise themselves with their medications and how to open the containers and packaging. They can discuss any needs or concerns, while the nurse has the opportunity to assess patient knowledge, evaluate previous teaching and identify those patients who will need ongoing support from the community services.

A programme of self-medication could help to reduce the number of drug errors, as it would incorporate extensive patient education and provide the opportunity for supervised practice of drug administration. Nurses reported that those patients who had self-medicated in hospital had a better understanding of all aspects of their drug regime (Bird 1990). Work by Scrivin and Bryant (1987) found that patients were very appreciative of a self-medication programme and medication errors reduced from 17.9% to 6.9% after the programme had been introduced. Also, if patients experience accidental overdoses it is safer for this to occur in hospital rather than the home environment.

Self-medication returns control to the patient, promoting comfort and demonstrating trust (Bird, 1990). A self-medicating patient will not be woken at 6 a.m., or stay awake until after midnight for sedation, or seek out a nurse for analgesia. Corrigon (1989) found that patients would question if the tablets looked different and were likely to refuse steroids until after breakfast. Webb (1990) found that most patients took in the process of self-medication very quickly, felt unrushed over administration and enjoyed having something positive to do. An 84-year-old patient stated, 'It's a good idea. I've achieved something – it gives me a bit of independence. I'm not stupid.'

Self-medication should provide a stimulus to reassess drug regimes and rationalise where appropriate. Bream (1985) identified patients who were taking all their pills at once rather than separately throughout the day. The safety and efficacy of a drug cannot be assessed until it is taken as instructed.

Stages in the implementation of self-medication

Planning

Planning is often considered the most important stage and cannot be rushed. It is vital to the overall success of the programme to gain the co-operation and support of all those involved including the ward staff, doctors and (crucially) the pharmacist.

Assessment

In some units assessment will be a dual process involving both the pharmacist and the nursing staff. The patients will be assessed on their understanding of the purpose of their medications, their safety in administration (i.e. timing and dosage), potential side effects to report and psychomotor skills in the handling and reading of their medications. It is at this stage that the nurse will enter into a thera-peutic partnership with the patient, offering support and education on an individualised basis to both the patient and their family as required. Table 2.10 lists the information that patients will require to know about their medications. An assessment document is often used to highlight any perceived problems and to determine the level of supervision required.

Table 2.10 What patients need to know about their medications (Quillagan 1990)

The name of the drug
How it is taken
Its intended actions
What dosage to take
The side effects
The time of the day it is to be given
How many tablets to take and how often
Whether to take it with food
How to obtain a repeat prescription
What to do if a dose is omitted
Check the expiry date
Not to stop essential medications without first consulting the doctor
Whether any special storage is required
Can you drive with them?
Not to take any non-prescription drug without first consulting the doctor

Accountability

Accountability can be a major concern to nurses when they consider implementing a self-medication programme. It can generate concerns of losing control over drug administration while still holding the same degree of responsibility. In fact, the nurse is not losing any element of control but is able to utilise the skills of educator, guide and supporter in a more constructive manner to ensure that patients are safely and knowledgeably administering their tablets. It could be argued that there are more concerns about accountability in the traditional system of drug administration, as nurses could be engaging in the provision of medicines without ascertaining the patient's knowledge and understanding of the therapy. Bird (1990) states that the problems that nurses anticipate – fear of patients forgetting to take their tablets, taking too many tablets or gaining access to other people's drugs – seldom occur in practice.

Implementation

In some units a staging process is used. The assessment process will determine the level the patients enter the programme and what degree of supervision is required, e.g.:

- level 1: the nurse administers the medicines, providing full explanation
- level 2: the patient administers the medicines with nurse supervision
- level 3: the patient administers the medicines without supervision (Sutherland et al. 1991).

Some areas have introduced memory aids in the form of calendar cards which have been shown to lead to fewer errors than written or verbal instructions (Wandless and Davie 1997).

Evaluation

Various degrees of supervision have been used, generally including at least daily discussions and observations of the patient's progress. Evaluation should include the obtainment of both the patient's and the nurse's views on progress.

Complementary medicine

Alternative and complementary medicine is the aggregate of diagnostic and therapeutic practices and systems that are separate from, and in contrast to, conventional scientific medicines (Champion 1994). Table 2.11 demonstrates the different types of complementary medicines currently available.

Table 2.11 Some complementary therapies

Acupuncture
Aromatherapy
Chinese medicine
Diet
Herbalism
Holistic medicine
Homeopathy
Massage
Naturopathy
Osteopathy
Reflexology
Spiritualism
Yoga

Diet

The extensive research into dietary treatments of rheumatoid arthritis has been reviewed by Buchanan et al. (1991); the results remain inconclusive. Individual dietary manipulation may be beneficial to selected patients (Panush et al. 1983, Darlington et al. 1986) but it is difficult to generalise from these findings and further study with sound methodological design is required.

Patients are extremely interested in this area and invest both time and money, striving to obtain relief from their symptoms. Dozens of publications vie with each other to suggest yet another method of ridding sufferers of pain and inflammation – often contradicting each other (ARC 1997). Trials have shown that the green lipped mussel extract (Seatone) does not work, but its sales continue (Champion 1994).

Surveys have found that many patients with rheumatoid arthritis consume diets that are marginally inadequate in several essential nutrients (Kowsari et al. 1983) (see Table 2.12). There is work to suggest that vitamin C, and perhaps vitamin E as an oxidant, could slow the progression of osteoarthritis (Champion 1994).

Rheumatoid arthritis is associated with moderate hypochromic normocytic anaemia, which is caused by a reduction in endogenous iron metabolism rather than dietary deficiency (Smith et al. 1985).

Table 2.12 Nutrients lacking in the diet of patients with rheumatoid arthritis

Calcium
Carbohydrates
Folacin
Magnesium
Pantothenic acid
Vitamin B_6
Vitamin D

Abnormalities in iron metabolism tend to be corrected as disease activity is suppressed.

Diets rich in fish oil containing N-3 fatty acids, along with a reduction of N-6 fatty acid intakes, have been associated with improvements in pain and stiffness. Some authors claim that fish oils will help inflammation by reducing arachidonic acid and leukotrienes production (Chaitow 1997). Dietary fish oils may prove to be more effective when used in combination with specific anti-inflammatory agents (Champion 1994).

Dietary advice for patients

For patients with osteoarthritis:

• reduce carbohydrates and fats
• keep weight down
• exercise regularly.

For patients with rheumatoid arthritis:

• eat a well balanced diet which contains minerals and vitamins
• eat more fruit and vegetables
• if weight loss is experienced, increase carbohydrate intake
• seek advice regarding drug therapy.

For patients with gout:

• advice on weight management
• reduction of high purine foods
• reduction in alcohol intake.

For patients with osteoporosis:

• (see Chapter 5.3).

Massage

Body massage is a method of manually manipulating the tissues of the body by either stroking, percussion or applying pressure. These actions increase the circulation of blood and lymph and induce relaxation by soothing sensory nerve endings in the skin (Goldberg 1991). There have been verbal reports from patients with rheumatoid arthritis and fibromyalgia that this form of intervention reduces pain and enhances sleep, but evaluation from a critical perspective remains limited.

Aromatherapy

Aromatherapy is the use of essential oils to promote healing in both a physical and psychological manner. Methods of application include massage, bathing, compresses and steam inhalations. Aromatherapy professes to provide pain relief, reduce inflammation and maintain joint mobility in patients with rheumatoid arthritis (Worwood 1993). Advice must be sought from a qualified aromatherapist before treatment can be instigated.

Reflexology

Reflexology is a form of massage applied to the reflex areas present in both the feet and hands. It is suggested that these reflex areas correspond with a specific area of the body and can stimulate the natural healing powers of the body (Dougans and Ellis 1992).

Reflex areas suggested to ease the symptoms of rheumatoid arthritis include:

- *diaphragm:* to reduce muscle tension
- *shoulder and arm:* to enhance circulation and nerve conduction
- *hip and leg:* to aid healing
- *spine:* to improve flexibility and to balance the nervous system
- *solar plexus:* to promote deep breathing and relaxation
- *parathyroid glands:* to maintain homeostasis with both calcium and potassium levels
- *liver:* to remove toxins from the body
- *adrenals:* to stimulate cortisone production, maintain mineral balance and enhance muscle tone (Norman 1992)

Acupuncture

Acupuncture is believed to change the vital energy which flows in the body and connects the internal organs with the superficial parts of the body (Beinfield and Korngold 1992). It is currently used for musculoskeletal conditions by orthodox, complementary and alternative practitioners (Champion 1994).

Herbal medicine

Herbal derivatives are widely used in orthodox rheumatology (Champion 1994), e.g.

• salicylates (willow bark)
• colchicine (autumn crocus)
• opiates (opium poppy)
• quinine (cinchona bark).

Controlled trials of other herbal treatments have proved inconclusive. Herbal preparations may be taken as tablets, infusions – as tea, tinctures or applied to baths. Popular herbs for rheumatism include aloe vera, comfrey, devil's claw, feverfew and evening primrose oil.

Naturopathy

This is a mixture of traditional folk wisdom, empiricism and selections of biomedical science. The basic principles (Champion 1994) are:

• the healing power of nature is fundamental
• treat the cause rather than the effect
• ill health results from a lowering of resistance due to diet, stress, etc.
• holism.

Treatment involves a combination of counselling, nutritional advice, herbal medicine and homeopathy remedies.

Appendix: Guidelines for nurses on the use and administration of intra-articular injections

What is an expanded role?

Role extension refers to nurses carrying out tasks not included in their normal training for registration. Most of these tasks relate to medical technical interventions usually carried out by doctors (Wright 1995).

Accountability

The *Scope of Professional Practice* (UKCC 1992) acknowledges that nurses are involved in negotiating the boundaries of practice and should be responsive to the needs of patients and clients. The onus is on individual nurses to recognise their own level of competence and decline any duties or responsibilities unless they are able to perform them in a safe and skilled manner. Nurses are also accountable for maintaining and improving their knowledge and should be familiar with the contents of the following documents:

Exercising Accountability (UKCC 1989)
Scope of Professional Practice (UKCC 1992)
Code of Professional Practice (UKCC 1992)
Standards for the Administration of Medicine (UKCC 1992)

What are intra-articular injections?

These are injections into the synovial joints. Long acting steroids are generally used for joint injections; hydrocortisone is used for soft tissue injections.

Indications for joint injections

Indications include:

- relief of pain from localised inflammation of the joint (e.g. rheumatoid arthritis)
- relief of pain from soft tissue discomfort
- to aid mobilisation
- to assist with rehabilitation (e.g. physiotherapy)
- to improve function.

Contraindications of joint injections

Contraindications include:

- local infection
- intra-articular fracture
- anticoagulant therapy
- bleeding disorders.

Preparation the nurse must undertake prior to the administration of intra-articular injections

The nurse must be able to demonstrate evidence of competency in the administration of intra-articular injections in accordance with the *Scope of Professional Practice* (UKCC 1992).

- Evidence of competency should indicate that the nurse has knowledge of:
  - anatomy and physiology of the joints and soft tissues
  - drugs used and their effects and side effects
  - indications and contra-indications for intra-articular injections
  - potential complications
  - aspiration and injection technique.
- Evidence of assessment of competency should be available.

- The employer must have precise knowledge of the employee's activities, and agree to them being undertaken by the employee (in accordance with vicarious liability).

The nurses's responsibility when giving intra-articular injections

- Obtain written instructions from the prescribing clinician detailing the drug, dosage and site of administration.
- Ensure the patient has given informed consent.
- Use an aseptic or no-touch technique.
- Aspirate the joint if swollen.
- Send a sample of synovial fluid for culture if it is very opaque, green or foul smelling.
- If no obvious signs of infection or contra-indications are present, administer the prescribed drug into the site stated.
- Document the drug, dosage and site of administration in the care records.
- Provide the patient with after care advice.

After care advice

The nurse must advise patients that:

- The joint may be painful for 24 hours after the injection. Take analgesia if necessary.
- It may take several days before benefit is felt.
- The injected joint should be rested as much as possible 24–48 hours after the injection.
- Short term facial flushing may be experienced.
- Localised skin atrophy may occasionally occur.
- To contact the Rheumatology Department if the patient has any concerns

Potential complications following the administration of intra-articular injections

Potential complications include:

- infections
- damage to the articular cartilage
- tendon rupture
- skin atrophy.

References

ARC (1997) Diet and arthritis: the facts. Arthritis Research Campaign. Arthritis Today 101: 4–5.

Austin HA, Klippel JH, Barlow JE et al (1986) Therapy of lupus nephritis: controlled trial of prednisolone and cytotoxic drugs. New England Journal of Medicine 314: 614–19.

Bagley CMJ, Bostick FW, De Vita VT (1973) Clinical pharmacology of cyclophosphamide. Cancer Research 33: 226–33.

Beardsley R, Anderson Johnson C, Kabat H (1983) A drug self administration programme. A behavioural appproach to patient education. Contemporary Pharmacy Practice 5(3): 156–60.

Beinfield H, Korngold E (1992) Between Heaven and Earth: A guide to Chinese Medicine. New York: Ballantine.

Bersani-Amado CA, Duarte AJ das, Tanji MM et al (1990) Comparative study of adjuvant induced arthritis in susceptible and resistant strains of rats. Analysis of lymphocyte sub populations. Journal of rheumatology 17: 153–8.

Bird C (1990) Patient Self Medication. Medicine Group UK. pp. 22–6.

Blocka K, Frust DE, Landaw E et al (1982) Single dose pharmacokinetics of auranofin in rheumatoid arthritis. Journal of rheumatology 9 (Suppl 8): 110–19.

Borel JF, Fever C, Gubler Hu, Stahelin H (1976) Biologic effects of cyclosporin A: A new antilymphocyte agent. Agents and Actions 6: 468–75.

Breedveld FC (1997) Future treatment In: Wolfe AD, Van Riel PLCM (eds) Early Rheumatoid Arthritis. Baillière's Clinical rheumatology. London: Baillière Tindall.

Brooks PM (1990) Slow acting anti-rheumatic drugs and immunosuppressives. Baillière's Clinical Rheumatology. London: Baillière Tindall.

Brooks PM (1994) Non steroidal anti-inflammatory drugs. In: Klippel J and Dieppe P (eds) Rheumatology. London: Mosby Year-Book Europe.

Brown RS, Bottomley WK (1990) The utilisation and mechanism of action of antidepressants in the treatment of chronic facial pain – a review of the literature. Anaesthetic Programme 37: 223–9.

Buchanan HM, Preston SJ, Brooks PM, Buchanan WW (1991) Is diet important in rheumatoid arthritis? British Journal of Rheumatology 30: 125–34.

Chaitow AL (1997) Diet for arthritis and rheumatism. International Journal of Alternative and Complementary medicine 15(4): 29–32.

Champion GD (1994) Proven remedies, alternative and complimentary medicine. In Klippel J and Dieppe P (eds) Rheumatology. London: Mosby Year-Book Europe.

Champion GD, Graham GC, Ziegler JB (1990) The gold complexes In: Brooks PM(ed.) Slow acting anti-rheumatic drugs and immunosuppressives. Baillière's clinical rheumatology. London: Baillière Tindall.

Christiansen C, Krane S (1993) Advances in Corticosteroids: A Seminar in print. Langhorne, USA: Adis International.

Choy EHS, Kingsley G, Corkhill MM, Panayi GS (1993) Intramuscular methylprednisolone is superior to pulse oral methylprednisolone during the induction phase of chrysotherapy. British Journal of Rheumatology 32: 734–9.

Clarke JH, Fitzgerald JF (1984) Effects of exogenous corticosteroid therapy on growth in children with HBs A gnegative chronic aggressive hepatitis. Journal of Pediatric Gastroenterology and Nutrition 3: 72–6.

Cohen ML (1994) Principles of pain and pain management. In: Klippel J, Dieppe P (eds) Rheumatology. London: Mosby Year-Book: Europe.

Cooper C, Kirwan JR (1990) The risk of local and systemic corticosteroid administration Baillière's Clinical Rheumatology 4: 305–32.

Corrigan MS (1989) Primary pharmacy. A patient self help service. Pharmaceutical Journal, October, 458–460.

Currey HLF (1988) Acute monoarthritis differential diagnosis and management. Collected reports on the rheumatic diseases. Chesterfield: Arthritis Research Campaign.

Darlington LG, Ramsey NW, Mansfield JR (1986) Placebo-controlled blind study of dietary manipulation therapy in rheumatoid arthritis. Lancet 1 (8475): 236–8.

Day R (1994) Pharmacologic approaches: SAARD I In: Klippel J, Dieppe P (eds) Rheumatology. London: Mosby Year Book Europe.

Del Pozo E, Graeber M, Elford P, Payne T (1990) Regression of bone and cartilage loss in adjuvant arthritis rats after treatment with cyclosporin A. Arthritis and Rheumatism 33: 247–52.

Deodhar AA, Brabyn J, Jones PW et al. (1995) Longitudinal study of hard bone densitometry in rheumatoid arthritis. Arthritis and Rheumatology (Suppl. 41): D183.

Dixon R, Christy N (1980) On the various forms of corticosteroid withdrawal syndrome. American Journal of Medicine 68: 224–30.

Donnelly S, Scott DL, Emery P (1992) The long term outcome and justification for early treatment. In: Emery P (ed) Management of early Inflammatory arthritis. Baillière's Clinical Rheumatology. London: Baillière Tindall.

Dougans I, Ellis S (1992) The art of Reflexology. Bath: Bath Press.

Easterbrook M (1988).Ocular effects and safety of anti-malarial agents. American Journal of Medicine 85 (Suppl 4A): 23–9.

Edwards C, Boucher I (1991) Davidson's Principles and Practice of Medicines. Edinburgh: Churchill Livingstone.

Elliot MJ, Maini RM, Feldmann M et al. (1994) Randomised double-blind comparison of chimeric menoclonal antibody to tumour necrosis factor (cA2) versus placebo in rheumatoid arthritis. Lancet 344: 1104–10.

Emmerson BT (1994) Antihyperuricemics In: Klippel J, Dieppe P (eds) Rheumatology. London: Mosby Year-Book Europe.

Eraker SA, Kirscht JP, Becher MH (1984) Understanding and improving patient compliance. Annals of Internal Medicine 100: 258–68.

Evans I, Spelman M (1983) The problem of non-compliancy with drug therapy. Drugs 25: 163–76.

Ferrante FM (1983) Opioids. In Ferrante FM, Vade Boncoeur TR (eds) Post Operative Pain Management. New York: Churchill Livingstone.

Flowers R (1996) The role of Cox 1 and Cox 2 – Implications for NSAID development. Current Opinions in Rheumatology 9(1): 15–19.

Fordham M (1986) Psychophysiological pain theories. Nursing 10(3): 360–4.

Fuller PL, Funder JW (1976) Mineralocorticoid and glucocorticoid receptors in human kidney. Kidney International 10: 154–7.

Furst PE, Clements PJ (1994) Pharmacologic approaches. SAARD II. In Klippel J, Dieppe P (eds) Rheumatology. London: Mosby Year-Book Europe.

George E, Kirwan JR (1990) Corticosteroid therapy in RA. Baillière's Clinical Rheumatology 4: 621–47.

Gibson H (1994) Psychology of Pain and Anaesthesia. London: Chapman & Hall.

Gibson T (1988) The treatment of gout: a personal view. Collected reports on the rheumatic diseases. Chesterfield: Arthritis Research Campaign.

Godschalk MF, Downs RW (1988) Effect of short term glucocorticoids on serum osteocalcin in healthy young men. Journal of Bone and Mineral Research 3: 113–15.

Goldberg AG (1991) Body Massage, 2nd edn. London: Redwood Press.

Goodwin JS, Regan M (1982) Cognitive dysfunction associated with Naproxen and Ibuprofen in the elderly. Arthritis and Rheumatism 25: 1013–15.

Guest G, Broyer M (1991) Alternate day corticosteroid therapy and growth in renal transplant patients. Annales de Pediatrie 38: 401–4.

Guyton AC (1991) Medical Physiology. London: WB Saunders.

Haagsma C, van de Putte L, van Riel R (1995) Sulfasalazine, Methotrexate and the combination in early RA, a double blinded randomised study. Arthritis and Rheumatism 36: 1501–9.

Hart D, Klinenberg J (1985) Choosing NSAID therapy. London: Adis Press.

Hill J, Bird HA, Hopkins R, Lawton C, Wright V (1991) The development and use of a patient knowledge questionnaire in RA. British Journal of Rheumatology 30: 45–9.

Hopkins R (1990) Sans awareness. Nursing Times 86(30): 50–1.

Huskisson EC, Woolf PC, Bourne HW, Scott J, Franklyn S (1974) Four anti-inflammatory drugs – responses and variations. British Medical Journal 1: 1084–9.

Jackson A (1995) Acute pain: its physiology and the pharmacology of analgesia. Nursing Times 91(16): 27–8.

Jamison RM (1996) Comprehensive pre-treatment and outcome assessment for chronic opioid therapy. Journal of Pain Symptom Management 11: 231–41.

Johnson L, Giles R (1993) Prescription for change. Nursing Times 89: 42–5.

Jones A (1997) Pain and its perception. Topical review series 3(10). Chesterfield: Arthritis Research Campaign.

Jordan S (1992) Drugs update: drugs for severe pain. Nursing Times 88(2): 24–7.

Joyce DA (1990) D-Penicillamine. In: Brookes PM (Ed.) Slow acting anti-rheumatic drugs and immunosuppressives. Baillière's clinical rheumatology. London: Baillière Tindall.

Karsh J, Klippel JH, Plotz Ph, Decker JL, Wright DG, Flye MW (1981) Lymphapheresis in RA. Arthritis and Rheumatism 24: 867–76.

Kennedy B (1981) Self medication. Canadian Nurse 77: 366–7.

Kirwan JR (1994) Systemic corticosteroids in rheumatology. In: Klippel JH, Dieppe P (eds.). Rheumatology. London: Mosby Year-Book Europe.

Kirwan JR and the Arthritis and Rheumatism Council Low Dose Glucocorticoid Study Group (1995) The effects of glucocorticoid steroid on joint destruction in RA. New England Journal of Medicine 333: 142–6.

Kowal A, Carstens Jr JH, Schinitzer TJ (1990). Cyclosporin in RA. In: Furst DE, Wenblatt ME (eds). Immunomodulators in the rheumatic diseases. New York: Marcel Dekker.

Kowsari B, Finnie SK, Carter RL et al. (1983) Assessment of the diet of patients with rheumatoid arthritis and osteoarthritis. Journal of American Dietary Association 82(6): 657–9.

Laurence D, Bennett P, Brown M (1997) Clinical Pharmacology. London: Churchill Livingstone.

Loeb J (1976) Corticosteroids and growth. New England Journal of Medicine 295: 547–42.

Lubkin IM (1990) Chronic Illness – Impact and Interactions. London:Jones and Bartlett.

Luqmani RA, Palmer RG, Bacon PA (1990) Azathioprine, cyclophosphamide and chlorambucil. In Brookes PM (ed.) Slow acting anti-rheumatic drugs and immunosuppressives. Baillièreís Clinical Rheumatology. London: Baillière Tindall.

Melzack R, Wall PD (1982) The Challenge of Pain. New York: Basic Books.

Miller TE, North DK (1981) Clinical injections, antibiotics and immunosuppression – a puzzling relationship (Editorial). American Journal of Medicine 71: 334–6.

Moll JM (1983) Management of Rheumatic Disorders. London: Chapman & Hall.

Mouridsen HT, Jacobsen E (1975) Pharmacokinetics of cyclophosphamide in renal failure. Acta Pharmacologica et Toxicologica 36: 409–14.

Newman S, Fitzpatrick R, Revensen T, Skinington S, Williams G (1996) Understanding RA. London: Routledge.

Norman L (1992) The Reflexology Handbook. Bath: Bath Press.

Nusslein HG, Herbst M, Manager BJ et al (1985) Total lymphoid irradiation in patients with refractory RA. Arthritis and Rheumatism 28: 1205–10.

Panush RS, Carter RL, Katz P, Kowarski B, Longley S, Finnie S (1983) Diet therapy for RA. Arthritis and Rheumatism 26(4): 462–71.

Parkin DM, Henney CR, Quirk J, Crooks J (1976) Deviation from prescribed drug treatment after discharge from hospital. British Medical Journal 1: 359–69.

Paulus HE, Machlide HI, Levine S et al (1977) Lymophocyte involvement in RA – studies during thoratic duct drainage. Arthritis and Rheumatism 24: 867–73.

Pearce S, Wardle J (1989) The practice of behavioural medicine. Oxford: Oxford University Press.

Piper JM, Ray WA, Doughery JR, Griffin MR (1991) Corticosteroid use and peptic ulcer role of NSAIDs. Annals of Internal medicine 114: 735–40.

Polito C, Oporto MR, Totino SF, La Manna D, Di Toro R (1986) Normal growth of nephrotic children during long term alternate day Prednisolone therapy. Acta Paediatrica Scandinavica 75: 245–50.

Porter DR, Capell HA (1990) The use of sulphasalazine as a disease modifying anti-rheumatic drug. In Brooks PM (ed.) Slow acting anti-rheumatic drugs and immuno-suppressives. Baillière's Clinical Rheumatology. London: Baillière Tindall.

Quilligan S (1990) When should you take your tablets? Professional Nurse September 639-640.

Reid IR, Chapman GE, Fraser TRC et al. (1986) Low serum osteocalcin levels in gluco-corticosteroid-treated asthmatics. Journal of Clinical and Endocrinological Metabolism 62: 379–383.

Rowbotham D (1993) Postoperative pain. Prescribers Journal 33(6): 237–43.

Schlegel S (1987) General characteristics of NSAIDs In: Paulus H, Furst D, Dromgoole S (eds.) Drugs for rheumatic diseases. New York: Churchill Livingstone.

Schwarzer AC, Arnold MH, Brooks PM (1990) Combination Therapy in RA. In: Brooks PM (ed.) Slow acting anti-rheumatic drugs and immunosuppressives. Baillière's Clinical Rheumatology. London: Baillière Tindall.

Scriven L, Bryan L (1987) Self medication on a surgical ward. New Zealand Nurse Journal 81: 25–6.

Smith J, Driscoll P, Coniff R (1985) Rheumatology Nursing – A Problem Orientated Approach. Chichester: John Wiley.

Songsiridej N, Furst DE (1990) Methotrexate – the rapidly acting drugs. In Brookes PM (ed.) Slow acting anti-rheumatic drugs and Immunosuppressives Baillière's Clinical Rheumatology. London: Baillière Tindall.

Speight TM (1987) Avery's drug treatment. Edinburgh: Churchill Livingstone.

Stewart RB, Cliff LE (1977) A review of medication errors and compliancy in ambulant patients. Clinical Pharmacy and Therapeutics 13: 463.

Stein C (1991) Peripheral analgesic effects of opioids. Pain System Management 6: 119–24.

Sutherland K, Morgan J, Sample S (1991) Self administering drugs – an introduction. Nursing Times 23: 29–33.

Thompson P, Dunne C (1995) NSAIDs – use and abuse. Collected Reports on Rheumatic Diseases. Chesterfield: Arthritis and Rheumatism Council.

Trouce J, Gould D (1990) Clinical Pharmacology for Nurses. London: Churchill Livingstone.

Turk DC, Melzac R, (1992) Handbook of Pain Assessment. New York: Guildford.

Turk JL, Parker D (1979) The effect of Cyclophosphamide on the immune response. Journal of Immunopharmacy 1: 127–37.

UKCC (1992) The Scope of Professional Practice. London: United Kingdom Central Council for Nursing, Midwifery and Health Visiting.

UKCC (1989) Exercising Accountability. London: United Kingdom Central Council for Nursing, Midwifery and Health Visiting.

Walker G (1994) ABPI Data Sheet Compendium. London: Datapharm Publications.

Watson CPN (1994) Anti-depressant drugs as adjuvant analgesia. Journal of Pain Symptom Management 9: 392–401.

Wandless I, Davie JW (1997) Can drug compliance in the elderly be improved? British Medical Journal 1: 359–61.

Webb C (1990) Self medication for elderly patients. Nursing Times 86(16): 46–9.

Weusten BLAM, Jacobs JWG, Bijlsma JWJ (1993) Corticosteroid pulse therapy in active RA. Seminars Arthritis and Rheumatism 23: 183–92.

Wilder RL, Decker JL (1983) T induced lymphocytes, leukapheresis and the pathogenesis of RA. Clinical and Experimental Rheumatology 1: 89–91.

Woolf CJ (1994) The dorsal horn state. Dependent sensory processing and the generation of pain In: Wall PD, Melzack R (Ed) Textbook of Pain. Edinburgh: Churchill Livingstone.

Worwood VA (1993) The fragrant Pharmacy. London: Bantam books.

Wright S (1995) The role of the nurse: extended or expanded? Nursing Standard 9(33): 25–9.

Yocum DE, Allen JB, Wahl Sm et al (1986) Inhibition by Cyclosporin A of streptococcal cell wall induced arthritis and hepatic granulomas in rats. Arthritis and Rheumatism 29: 262–73.

Further reading

Doherty M et al. (1992) Rheumatology Examination and Injection Techniques. Doherty M, Hazelman BL, Hutton CW, Perry DJ (eds). London: WB Saunders.

Klippel JH, Dieppe PA (1995) Practical Rheumatology. London: Mosby Year-Book Europe.

Part 3
The role of the rheumatology nurse

SARAH RYAN

Learning objectives

After reading the chapters in Part 3 you should be able to:

- Describe the philosophy that underpins rheumatology nursing
- Explain the role of the nurse in preparing the patient to commence a DMARD
- Discuss the initial and ongoing drug monitoring and support the patient requires
- Demonstrate an understanding of the safety monitoring required in the surveillance of DMARDs.

3.1 Therapeutic relationship in rheumatology nursing

Patients with inflammatory arthritis, such as rheumatoid arthritis, can experience a range of physical, psychological, social and/or sexual problems. The role of the nurse is to support, guide, educate and empower the patient and their family so that problems can be identified and care that has meaning and relevance for the patient can be implemented. This has to be a shared process between the patient and the nurse, because conditions such as rheumatoid arthritis are not curable and the patient must be committed to a long-term treatment plan. Patients with disease activity (determined by haematological and biochemical markers, radiography results and clinical findings) will require a combination of drug therapy to reduce symptoms such as pain and stiffness and also to suppress the condition, minimising the potential harm that prolonged inflammation can cause. Analgesia and non-steroidal anti-inflammatory drugs (NSAIDs) can provide symptoms relief and the disease-modifying antirheumatic drugs DMARDs (see Table 3.1) can suppress disease activity. The nurse requires in-depth knowledge of the condition and treatment options, and needs to employ the skills of educator to provide the patient with sufficient information to contribute to shared decision-making before the commencement of drug therapy.

What is rheumatology nursing?

Therapeutic nursing has been defined by Powell (1991) as that practice where the nurse has made a difference to the health state of the patient or client, and where the nurse is aware of how and why this positive difference has occurred. Levine (1973) distinguishes between nursing which is *supportive* in nature – seeking to

149

Table 3.1 Disease-modifying antirheumatic drugs (DMARDs)

Auranofin
Azathioprine
Cyclophosphamide
Cyclosporin
Dapsone
Gold injections
Hydroxychloroquine/chloroquine
Methotrexate
Minocyline
Penicillamine
Phenylbutazone
Sulphasalazine

prevent further deterioration – and that which is *therapeutic* – promoting adaptation and contributing to the restoration of well-being. The introduction of drug therapy in conjunction with other treatment interventions such as exercise can be seen as fulfilling both a supportive and a therapeutic role, preventing deterioration and leading to an improvement in symptoms and thereby enabling the patient to participate more fully in meaningful life activities.

Caring is the most important value of rheumatology nursing. Although it is often referred to as a basic requirement, there is nothing basic about high quality nursing care which requires a combination of knowledge, understanding and expertise. Caring involves both an *action element*, identifying and meeting the needs of the patient, and an *emotional element* which involves having regard for people as individuals and being concerned about what happens to them (Malin and Teasdale 1991). It appears that in many situations the action element remains the dominant feature of nursing practice, where interactions with patients are governed by their physical care needs, resulting in the neglect of their emotional needs (Henderson 1994). Yet we know that from the patient's perspective it is how the individual nurse relates to the patient – the emotional style – that determines whether a patient perceives a care episode as satisfactory or not (Smith 1988). For care to be effective and holistic in nature, the nurse must incorporate both the action element and the emotional element into care delivery. The adoption of this approach is as important in the instigation of drug therapy as in all treatment interventions, as the patient will have to be satisfied on an emotional level as to the value of drug therapy for compliance to occur.

Nurse–patient relationship

The most important element in rheumatology nursing is the relationship that exists between the patient and the nurse. Such a relationship requires both time and knowledge allowing the nurse to begin to empower the patient so that an informed decision regarding care management can be reached. The relationship needs to be founded on participation. There is the assumption that by involving the patients in their own care they will ultimately obtain the status of participants, but it may well be that the patients are participating from the nurse's frame of reference, rather than from their own viewpoint. Asking the patients to write down their expectations regarding drug therapy may provide the starting point from which the partnership can commence.

Some factors needed for a therapeutic relationship

Genuine participation. It is important to encourage the patients to participate in as many treatment decisions as possible. When patients chooses a course of action, such as commencing sulphasalazine, they are more likely to adhere even if the beneficial effects take some time to emerge, which in the case of this particular drug could be anything from 2 to 4 months. Informing the patients about different drug options and enabling the patients to choose from them should heighten their sense of control.

Exploration of lay beliefs. Until the nurse has spent time exploring the patients' own beliefs about the purpose and outcome of drug therapy it will not be possible to arrive at shared treatment objectives.

Establishment of realistic goals. Trying to reach unrealistic goals will only demoralise and adversely affect self-esteem. If the patients are not informed that DMARDs take many months before benefit can be assessed they could become disillusioned with the treatment if symptoms did not improve after the first few weeks and discontinue the regime.

Provision of information specific to the individuals' situation. It is not helpful to be given generalised information and told, for example, what percentage of patients respond well to gold treatment. The individuals require information that is holistic and relevant to their own particular situation.

Involvement of significant others. It is important that family members are included and assist in care planning so that care options decided on can be endorsed and implemented within the patients' supportive framework and within their own social setting.

Maintaining contact. It is important that the patient has access to a knowledgeable practitioner who is familiar with their care, at any time when there is a perceived change in disease activity or self-management. This can be maintained through a telephone helpline system which provide the patients with a designated point of contact and help to reduce anxiety and provide support.

Telephone helpline

Many rheumatology nurses are involved in operating a telephone helpline service for patients. An unpublished annual audit of the helpline at the Staffordshire Rheumatology Centre revealed that the most frequent usage related to DMARD therapy. Through the helpline the nurse is able to provide advice directly to the individual concerned and co-ordinate further treatment if it is required, e.g. intra-articular injection or the commencement of a sulphasalazine desensitising regime if a rash occurs after the introduction of sulphasalazine therapy.

The telephone helpline also provides direct access for other members of the team involved in the patient's medical and nursing care to seek advice. For example, a GP may ring to question whether gold injections should be discontinued because of the slight presence of haematuria on a urinalysis dipstick test. The immediate advice by the nurse to continue can prevent treatment being stopped unnecessarily. It also enables a consistency of care management to develop between members of primary and secondary health care teams. This reinforces communication links and promotes a greater appreciation of the different roles of these two groups.

Philosophy of rheumatology nursing

A philosophy of practice is required to enable nurses within rheumatology to work as a united team with identified shared goals for patient management. A philosophy consists of a system of beliefs from which care practice evolves. The establishment of a philosophy has to include debate and discussion from all members of the nursing team. It is a statement of purpose and will require commitment from all concerned for it to be integrated into practice. If a shared approach to care is not adopted then disunity and fragmentation of care will occur. A rheumatology nursing philosophy of care can be divided into four main areas which are interlinked and complementary to each other. These include:

- health
- beliefs relating to the environment
- beliefs relating to the individual patient
- beliefs relating to nursing.

Health

Health is achieved when the patient is able to function on a physical, psychological and social level. This is not a reinstatement of complete wellbeing in all these spheres of life; rather, that the patient perceives that they are able to make a useful contribution to all areas of activity. Health requires adaptations and the development of coping strategies to minimise the symptoms of arthritis. It does not mean the removal of all symptoms, which would be an unrealistic outcome and an unfair burden to place on patients. Health and illness are not static entities: they vary, depending on:

- disease activity
- coping strategies
- available resources
- support.

Rheumatoid arthritis is characterised by flares and remissions of disease activity, and the patients may find themselves alternating between health and illness or functioning well on a physical level but not on a psychological level. The patients need to know how to access a knowledgeable nurse when they experience a stage in their condition that presents different or recurring problems, so that the situation can be reassessed collectively and necessary modifications made to the treatment programme.

Beliefs relating to the environment

A patient needs to be involved in the planning of all aspect of care to feel committed and able to implement the agreed treatment programme based on the individuals' perceived needs (Tones 1991), and this applies equally to drug therapy. Neglect of individual concerns can lead to non-adherence with treatment. Nurses need to identify any existing internal and external barriers. Patients may not be able to open their medication container owing to reduced manual dexterity, or be afraid to continue with treatment owing to adverse peer pressure. If the orientation of the consultation between the nurse and the patient does not encourage shared discussion, the patients may not feel part of the treatment regime and may discontinue their medications if they are not immediately effective.

Beliefs relating to the individual patients

The individuals' lay beliefs must be explored before any treatment plan is decided so that the care programme that emerges has both relevance and meaning for the individuals concerned. Lay beliefs are usually consistent over time and pertinent to the individual concerned (Donovan 1991). If patients have in their lay belief system the thought that drug treatment such as gold has the potential for only damaging side effects to occur and not the potential for improvement, they may reject it as a treatment option. The patients will require explanation of the disease process before they can understand the role of drug therapy. If they do not understand that their pain, stiffness and fatigue is related to disease activity they may be not perceive drug treatment as a useful adjunct to other therapy.

The individuals have a right to be an active not a passive recipient of care, so informed decisions can be made and the management of the condition viewed as a shared commitment between the patient and the health professional. Patients may not feel equipped to adapt to this role at first, but as the nurse begins to share knowledge with the patient and a therapeutic relationship develops, the patients may feel more able to contribute to care decisions.

Beliefs relating to nursing

The nurse is a knowledgeable practitioner, using evidence-based practice to underpin holistic care management and receiving support and commitment from service management to develop patient focused services such as drug monitoring clinics.

3.2 Role of the nurse in drug therapy

Empowerment

Once the clinical decision has been made to commence a patient on DMARD therapy, the patient will require time with a knowledgeable practitioner so that the following aspects can be discussed:

- purpose of the medication
- dosage and time of administration
- potential side effects
- monitoring regime
- patients' expectations of treatment
- what to do if a problem arises.

Tones (1991) defines empowerment as the process whereby an individual or community of individuals acquires power, i.e. the capacity to control other people and resources. By having the particular drug therapy and the rationale for its introduction explained, the patient will begin to determine its acceptability from their particular viewpoint. Klein (1974) describes five categories of patient involvement:

1. *Information.* This is the process whereby the health professional gives the information to the patients and the patients passively receive it. This is not useful for commencing patients on drug therapy, as the patients are the individuals responsible for the administration of the medication and to comply with the proposed regime must be committed to the type of treatment being advocated. Patient–physician communication may be the single most important variable affecting adherence (Bradley

1989). For communication to be successful, the clinician must present information clearly, and the patients need to seek clarification and ensure that their concerns are addressed (Newman et al. 1996).

Factors that influence effective practitioner–patient communication include (Newman et al. 1996):

- The nature of the explanation concerning the diagnosis, the course and purpose of treatment. When rheumatologists were recorded as having made a clear statement about the purpose of the drug treatment 79% of patients were compliant with their therapy, compared to only 33% of patients when the explanation offered was not clear (Daltroy 1993).
- An overuse of medical jargon which excludes the patients from shared discussion.
- A shared agreement of the goals for treatment, which is essential. Arluke (1980) found that some patients with rheumatoid arthritis stopped their medication at the first sign of improvement because they held the belief that drug efficacy would reduce over time.
- The need to ascertain the patients' concerns regarding drug treatment. Several studies have shown that practitioners misperceive the patients' needs regarding the amount, content and preferred method for providing information (e.g. drug information sheets) on arthritis and its treatments (Potts et al. 1986).

2. *Consultation.* The health professional may consult the patients and may use the information gained. This will not in itself lead to a shared approach towards treatment management, as the practitioner may not have obtained the patients' beliefs, values and expectations which are all potent factors affecting adherence – not only because of their direct relationship to health behaviour but also because they are subject to misinterpretation unless clarification is sought and will ultimately influence how satisfied the patient is with the consultation.

3. *Negotiation.* Here equality exists and both parties contribute to the decision-making and negotiate the treatment. The nurse should begin by ascertaining the patients' concerns regarding treatment, and identify potential compliance difficulties and jointly plan how to overcome them (Daltroy 1993).

4. *Participation.* Patients' values are taken into account and underpin the decision process. Patients may prefer not to commence methotrexate if they enjoy a social drink, and will be more likely to comply with an alternative drug where they do not have to abstain from alcohol.

5. *Veto-participation.* The patients hold the right not to comply with treatment. Liang (1989) describes non-compliance as the ultimate experience of independence. If this occurs it should do so only after full negotiation has occurred, and not as a result of ignorance or non-disclosure. The nurse should seek to ascertain the reason why the patient has declined drug therapy. It may be due to a lack of knowledge or apprehensions that have not been discussed. If patients decline therapy they must be given the opportunity to reaccess the service at any time to reassess their condition and other treatment options.

Commencement of DMARDs: patient preparation

The mode of action of DMARDs has been discussed in depth in Chapter 2. Patients often commence DMARDs at a time when their arthritis is in an illness phase, with evidence of increased disease activity. This will often cause the patient to experience an increase in symptomatology inducing pain, stiffness, fatigue low mood and systemic manifestations such as anaemia. For most DMARDs, it takes many months before their ability to affect the disease process can be assessed, although drugs such as methotrexate do have the potential to work quicker. Patients respond at different rates to a combined treatment programme but will require education, support and guidance at the beginning of treatment and throughout. The nurse, in conjunction with the patient, will need to plan interventions to enable the patient to cope with increased symptomatology: this may include a combination of exercise, relaxation, pacing activities, review of analgesia or an inpatient stay.

The objectives of ongoing education and care provision are to enable patients to participate effectively in their own management, develop coping skills, make informed choices about their treatment and weigh up the consequences of their action or inaction. Lorig et al. (1987), in a comprehensive review of patient education studies, demonstrated positive improvement in patient knowledge, self-care beliefs, medication adjustment and compliance, as well as psychosocial characteristics such as anxiety, depression, self-esteem, locus of control and health status.

After patients have received a full explanation regarding the drug treatment proposed and has been given the opportunity to discuss concerns and expressed a commitment to the therapy, safety preparation may be necessary before commencement of the drug therapy.

For example, if a patient is to commence methotrexate, a chest radiograph is required. Patients with existing lung disorder may not be commenced on methotrexate because pneumonitis is a potential side effect. The radiograph provides a useful baseline with which later films can be compared should a breathing problem materialise. Patients must also commit themselves to the abstaining from alcohol owing to the action of methotrexate on the liver. All patients (male and female) beginning cytotoxic agents must be advised to take strict contraceptive precautions on starting the therapy, and continue for at least 6 months after the therapy is discontinued.

Monitoring clinics

Patients receiving DMARDs require regular safety monitoring of therapy and assessment of disease activity. This is usually carried out within the holistic framework of a nurse led follow-up clinic. The full functions of such clinics are set out in Table 3.2.

Table 3.2 Functions of a nurse-led clinic (Hill 1992)

Assessing the progress of the disease
Monitoring the progress of the disease
Monitoring drug response
Initiating and interpreting clinical and laboratory data
Acting as educator
Expert source of referral to other members of the multidisciplinary team
Research

Phelan et al. (1992) found that 86% of rheumatology nurse specialists were undertaking drug monitoring as part of their role. The nurse-led clinics allow partnership, intimacy and reciprocity to evolve between the nurse and the patients and provide the medium for an ongoing therapeutic partnership to develop in which the nurse will assess all care needs and identify problems that may require a referral to other members of the health care team, such as the chiropodist. The clinic also provides the forum for education and the development of coping strategies. The nurse's role evolves from supportive to therapeutic: instead of concentrating exclusively on preventing deterioration, the nurse will incorporate essential nursing functions (see Table 3.3) to promote adaptation to the condition for the patients and their families.

Table 3.3 Key nursing functions (Wilson Barnett 1984)

Understanding illness and treatment from the patient's viewpoint
Providing continuous psychological care during illness and critical events
Helping people cope with illness or potential health problems
Providing comfort
Co-ordinating treatment and other events affecting the patient

For care to be meaningful within an individual context, nurses must understand the impact of illness from the patient's viewpoint (Ryan 1996). The nurse must work actively with the patient to establish realistic achievable goals which incorporate the patients lay beliefs.

Operational workings of a drug monitoring clinic

Most patients receiving DMARDs and cytotoxic agents require weekly blood tests and in certain cases urinalysis for the first month of treatment. For most medications drug monitoring may then be continued at monthly intervals. Different units have different policies for the monitoring of drug therapy. There has been an attempt to standardise practice with the publication of guidelines from the British Society of Rheumatology, but most units appear to adhere to their own policies based on their own experience of treatment with these agents. Kay and Puller (1992) found marked variations amongst respondents in monitoring schedules and in the interpretation of results. For legal reasons it is necessary to be familiar with the data sheet recommendations. Table 3.4 details the monitoring regime in operation at the Staffordshire Rheumatology Centre.

At each weekly visit the patient is seen by the same rheumatology nurse to allow the continuation of the therapeutic relationship.

What the nurse does during the weekly visit

- Assess safety in administration, e.g. ensuring that D-Penicillamine is taken on an empty stomach to increase absorbency.
- Monitor and observe for any drug reactions that have occurred, e.g. gastrointestinal, skin, urinary abnormalities and chest manifestations.
- Take blood to ascertain any bone marrow suppression leading to a reduction in red blood cells, white blood cells and platelet count; elevation in liver function tests, creatinine levels and urea

Table 3.4 Monitoring regime for DMARDs at the Staffordshire Rheumatology Centre

Drug	Specific requirement
Auranofin	weekly urinalysis for 4 weeks, then monthly
Azathioprine	weekly liver function tests for 4 weeks, then monthly
Cyclophosphamide	weekly urea and electrolytes for 4 weeks then every 2–4 weeks depending on regime
Cyclosporin	weekly creatinine, blood pressure and urinalysis for 4 weeks, then monthly
Dapsone	haemoglobin after first week of treatment
Gold injections	weekly urinalysis
Methotrexate	weekly liver function tests for 4 weeks, then monthly
Minocyline	weekly liver function tests for 4 weeks, then monthly
D-Penicillamine	weekly urinalysis for 4 weeks, then monthly
Sulphasalazine	weekly liver function tests for 4 weeks, then monthly for 6 months, then 6-monthly

Generic requirement for all DMARDS: full blood count, erythrocyte sedimentation rate platelets; differentials weekly for the first month and then monthly.

and electrolytes where indicated. Hill's (1994) research demonstrated that the nurse practitioner is able to identify and instigate appropriate action from blood results.

- Provide the patient with time to discuss any perceived problems or concerns, e.g.
  - Is it safe to have vaccinations?
  - Is it normal to experience increased stiffness after the administration of intramuscular gold?
- Assess for evidence of increased disease activity, e.g. synovitis. This may necessitate a different treatment intervention e.g. the administration of intra- articular injections. Phelan et al. (1992) found that 12% of nurse specialists within rheumatology were engaged in the provision of intra-articular injections, and this number is rapidly increasing as nurses seek to develop their practice around patient need and provide a more comprehensive programme of care expansion and is in accordance with principles established in the scope of professional practice (UKCC 1992). This framework encourages and supports nurses to develop practice which has been shown to benefit patient care directly, as long as it does not fragment existing care or involve inappropriate delegation of duties. It would be inappropriate, indeed unsafe practice to develop one's role without first obtaining

the theoretical knowledge and practical expertise necessary to ensure understanding and safe practice. Benner (1984) states that an expert nurse requires a combination of academic achievement, recognised clinical expertise and practical experience.

- Access other care needs within a holistic framework (see Figure 3.1) and refer where appropriate to other member of the multidisciplinary team.
- Advise the patient of the telephone helpline, providing a designated point of contact with a knowledgeable practitioner should any problems or concerns arise before the next appointment.

Documentation

At the Staffordshire Rheumatology Centre the nurse-led monitor clinic has a computerised system which removes the need for medical or nursing notes. Kay (1989) states that more use could be made of computer technology in drug monitoring. All relevant information about the patient is entered on to the database. This includes demographic data, blood and urine results, clinical letters, medications taken and reasons for discontinuation where appropriate. The computer is programmed to alert the operator to any results that fall

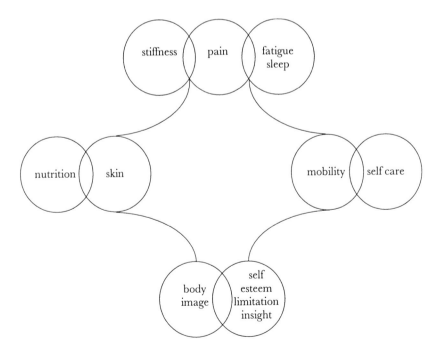

Figure 3.1 The rheumatology nursing forum problem model (Reproduced with permission of the Royal College of Nursing).

outside the normal parameters such as three consecutive falls in platelets. It is also an invaluable communication tool as any member of the nursing and medical team can place a message on the patient's computerised record that will be acknowledged by the nurse conducting the clinic. This may include requests for additional investigations to be made while the patient is in clinic so that they do not have the inconvenience of being recalled. Other units use a metrology graph which includes a visual analogue pain scale, early morning stiffness, articular index, grip strength and the recording of drug regimes. A list of past medication and the reasons for discontinuation is kept on the reverse of the graph for easy referral. Joint injections, intramuscular steroid injections, infusions, admissions, trauma and even domestic stress are recorded on the chart because they all have a bearing on disease activity. This method of documentation enables the course of the disease to be followed easily (Thompson et al. 1992).

Use of protocols

The establishment of protocols to guide decision-making and ensure continuing of care and safety in practice requires collaboration and commitment from all health professionals involved in the monitoring and assessment of drug therapy. They provide an educational tool for nurses by ensuring that practice is research based, and act as a dynamic framework updated when new evidence becomes available. The protocols may cover:

• urinary abnormalities
• gastrointestinal side effects
• skin manifestations
• chest symptoms
• alteration of drug dosages.

(This last point is in accordance with the Medicines Act of 1968 which states that no person shall administer, other than to himself any such medicinal products unless he/she is an appropriate practitioner or a person acting in accordance within the directions of an appropriate practitioner.)

Included in the Appendix are the protocols used for the daily drug monitoring clinic at the Staffordshire Rheumatology Centre. This provides an example of the framework we have adopted, enabling these protocols to be a fluid and dynamic tool supporting nurses in the decision-making process.

Having such a framework enables the nurse to take immediate action when faced with rare but serious side effects such as myasthenic symptoms as a consequence of D-Pencillamine therapy. Ryan (1997) states that during the first year of using such protocols over 800 patients were reviewed in the clinic with only 2% requiring medical referral. Before the instigation of the protocols 16% of patients were referred annually for a medical consultation primarily as a result of limitations being placed on nurse decision-making skills.

The protocols can also ensure continuity of care when the patient moves back into the community setting.

Conclusion

The role of the nurse in drug therapy for patients with a rheumatological condition is of major importance and indeed may be regarded as the most crucial component that determines whether patients comply successfully with their drug regimes. The purpose and full implications of commencing new therapy need to be explored fully by a knowledgeable practitioner, incorporating in this process the values, beliefs and expectations of patients and their families. This will enable the patient to be an active, not passive, recipient of treatment.

The nurse will develop a therapeutic relationship containing both an action and emotional element, based on a philosophy of rheumatology nursing that places patients' perceived care requirements at the centre of all care management programmes. It demands that the nurse has the necessary training and preparation in both academic understanding and clinical expertise so that care of that is safe, effective and holistic can be offered to all patients. The nurse needs to employ the skills of educator to guide and provide continuous support at a time of increased disease activity, so that the efficacy of drug therapy and its influence on the condition can be assessed accurately.

3.3 Investigations

Haematological investigations

The most frequently requested laboratory test is the full blood count (Higgins 1996). This test examines three groups of cells with different functions: platelets, red cells (erythrocytes) and white cells (leucocytes). Around 2–2.5 ml of venous blood is required in a tube containing an anticoagulant.

Red blood cells

Red blood cells (erythrocytes)are biconcave disks. Their main function is to transport haemoglobin around the body and supply oxygen to the tissues. The average number of red blood cells per cubic millimetre of blood is about 5 million. The number of red blood cells available in the circulation is regulated so that there is an adequate source to provide oxygenation of the tissues without stopping blood flow. The cell has a very flexible structure which allows it to alter shape as it passes through the capillaries without damage. Altitude and the degree of exercise undertaken can affect the number of circulating red blood cells. Red blood cells derive from a cell known as the *haemocytoblast* and are produced in the bone marrow.

Vitamin B_{12} (cyanocobalamin)

Vitamin B_{12} is a nutrient that is required for all cells of the body. An absence or reduced supply of vitamin B_{12} will severely hinder the rate of red blood cell production. The problem is often the failure to absorb vitamin B_{12} from the gastrointestinal tract, as occurs in pernicious anaemia. Gastric secretion contain a substance called the *intrinsic factor* which combines with the vitamin B_{12} in the food, so preparing it for absorption by the gut, but in pernicious anaemia the gastric muscosa does not secrete the intrinsic factor and therefore absorption cannot occur.

In the normal process vitamin B_{12} is stored in large quantities in the liver after absorption from the gastric system. The total amount of vitamin B_{12} required every day to assist in red blood cell production is less than 1 microgram and the store in the liver is 1000 times that amount.

Folic acid

Folic acid is part of the vitamin B complex, and deficiency of this can also hinder the production of red blood cells.

Anaemia

The typical anaemia of rheumatoid arthritis is a normocytic normochromic anaemia, the haemoglobin being around 10–12 g/dl. There appears to be a correlation between disease activity and the severity of anaemia. Some DMARDs (e.g. gold) may induce anaemia by attacking erythyroid progenitor cells but in other situations studies show that these therapies may normalise erythropiesis (Pincus et al. 1990)

The cause of anaemia in rheumatoid arthritis is multifactorial. Iron utilisation is impaired, as indicted by reduced serum iron and transferritin concentration. As with other forms of chronic inflammation there is an increased synthesis of ferritin and haemosiderin, abnormal retention of iron from red blood cells by the reticuloendothelial system and an increase of lactoferritin which contributes to the binding and lowering of serum iron (Matteson et al. 1994).

Anaemia means a deficiency of red blood cells, with haematocrit sometimes as low as 10%. The anaemia of rheumatoid arthritis can be complicated by:

• blood loss (NSAIDS can cause intestinal blood loss)
• poor nutrition
• intercurrent infections
• autoimmune haemolytic anaemia
• bone marrow suppression secondary to drug treatment, e.g. gold.

A macrocytic macrochromic anaemia may be due to vitamin B_{12} or folate deficiency, alcohol intake or the mechanisms of sulphasalazine or methotrexate.

White blood cells

When blood is stained and viewed under the microscope it is possible to identify five types of white blood cell (leucocyte). A full blood count measures their total number and and also counts the number of each of the five types. This is the *differential count*. The normal range of values and differential results can be seen in Table 3.5.

Table 3.5 White blood cells

		proportion of total (%)
total white blood cell count	$4-11 - 10^9/L$	100
neutrophils	$2.5-7.5 - 10^9/L$	40–75
lymphocytes	$1.5-4.0 - 10^9/L$	20–40
monocytes	$0.2-0.8 - 10^9/L$	2–10
eosinophils	$0.04-0.4 - 10^9/L$	1–6
basophils	$0.01-0.1 - 10^9/L$	<1

The white blood cells are the mobile units of the body's protective system. They are formed in the bone marrow and the lymph nodes before being transported in the blood to the different parts of the body where they are used. All white blood cells have a limited life span, and adequate numbers are maintained by marrow production.

White blood cells play a central role in the process of inflammation. The purpose of the inflammatory response is a complex integration of cellular function, and although each type of leucocyte has a different and well-defined function they operate in conjunction, communicating via a range of chemical messengers called *cytokines* (Higgins 1996).

Leucocytosis (a raised white blood cell count) occasionally occurs in rheumatoid arthritis but it is not a typical feature. If marked, it should raise suspicions of a superseded infection (either systemic or a septic arthritis) a postinfected arthritis or one of the varieties of polyarteritis.

Leucopenia (a reduced white blood cell count) can occur in systemic lupus erythematosus and in Felty's syndrome, but the commonest cause is the use of DMARDs.

Neutrophils

Between 40% and 75% of circulating white blood cell are neutrophils. They are the first line of defence against bacterial invasions. They are present in large numbers at the place of invasion, where they ingest and kill bacteria by a process of phagocytosis.

Monocytes

Monocytes are mobile white blood cells that filter out of the blood and into the tissues where they are referred to as *macrophages*. Their key role is probably as an antigen-presenting cell. Lymphocytes cannot respond to naked antigen; it must first be processed by and presented on the surface of an antigen-presenting cell. Macrophages become attached to tissues and remain attached for months, even years. They are involved in the primary clearance of highly resistant bacteria such as mycobacteria.

Monocytes manufacture a range of cytokines that attract or activate other cells involved in the inflammatory response, e.g. macrophages produce interleukin-1 which activates a type of lymphocyte to kill viruses (Oppenheim 1986).

Basophils

These are seen only rarely in peripheral blood. They mature in the tissues becoming mast cells. These cells liberate heparin into the blood to prevent blood coagulation and to assist in tissue repair. The mast cells also release histamine and small quantities of bradykinin and serotinin during inflammation.

Eosinophils

Eosinophils are natural phagocytes. They collect at the site of antigen-antibody reaction in the tissues and 'digest' the combined antigen-antibody complex after the immune process has performed its function. Esoinophils are involved in the pathogenesis of hypersensitivity (allergic) reactions. Their number is greatly increased in the circulating blood during allergic reactions.

Eosinophils accompanying rheumatoid arthritis are sometimes associated with extra-articular manifestations (Parrish et al. 1971). Although the pathogenesis is not known, immune complexes may be chemotactic for eosinophils (e.g. attracted towards the source of the chemical).

Eosinophilia has also been associated with high titre of rheuma-toid factor, elevation of serum gammaglobulins and diminished serum complement levels (Matteson et al. 1994). Pulmonary compli-cations may be associated with eosinophilia (Crisp et al. 1982), or it may be associated with drug therapy such as gold.

Lymphocytes

Between 20% and 40% of circulating white blood cells are lympho-cytes, which are the cells of the acquired immune system. Although a routine blood count cannot differentiate between them, there are two types – B lymphocytes and T lymphocytes. *B lymphocytes* produce antibodies and *T lymphocytes* are responsible for the elimi-nation of viruses and other micro-organisms that infect the cell of the host and are not 'visible' for antibody attack (Higgins 1996). The two types of lymphocyte function are independent, and a normal immune response requires adequate numbers of both B and T lymphocytes.

Causes of low white cell count

A low white blood cell count is significant because it indicates a reduction of the body's protection against infection. If the neutrophil count falls below 0.5×10^9, patients are likely to become susceptible to frequently recurring bacterial infections. If levels drop further, life is threatened by the risk of overwhelming infection.

Causes of leucopenia include:

- Felty's syndrome
- Aplastic anaemia (A pancytopenia where reduced production of bone marrow stem cells results in reduced number of red cells, white cells and platelets. Aplastic anaemia can be inherited, as can pancytopenia, although most causes of the latter arise as side effects of cytotoxic drugs.)
- Systemic lupus erythematosus.
- Side effect of DMARDs, e.g. D-Penicillamine
- Leukaemia (This is associated with a reduced neutrophil count because bone marrow production of large numbers of abnormal immature white cells continues at the expense of normal white cell production.)
- AIDS
- Hodgkin's disease.

Agranulocytosis

The bone marrow stops producing white blood cells, leaving the body unprotected against bacteria and other agents that might invade the tissues. Within 2 days of production ceasing, ulcers appear in the mouth and colon and severe respiratory infection develops. Bacteria then rapidly invade the surrounding tissues and the blood; without treatment, death usually occurs within a week.

Platelets

The number of platelets in each cubic millimetre of blood is normally around 300 000. An increased amount of platelets (*thrombocytosis*) is a frequent finding in active rheumatoid arthritis and may well correlate with the number of joints involved, the amount of active synovitis and the presence of extra-articular features. The mechanism of thrombocytosis is uncertain; an increase in the intravascular coagulation with a compensatory increase in platelet production has been suggested (Matteson et al. 1994). The thrombocytosis does not predispose to an increase in thrombotic events and is not correlated with bone marrow neoplastic changes. A reduced platelet count (*thrombocytopenia*) is rare in rheumatoid arthritis except when related to drug treatment or Felty's syndrome.

Biochemical investigations

Hepatic function

Liver function abnormalities may reflect the anaemia, thrombocytosis and increased erythrocyte sedimentation rate of active inflammatory disease such as rheumatoid arthritis. Examination of liver histology at this time reveals only minimal non-specific change and some periportal mononuclear cell infiltration (Matteson et al. 1994).

Active rheumatoid arthritis may be associated with an increase in liver enzymes especially serum glutamic oxaloacetic transaminase (SGOT) and alkaline phosphatase (Fernandes et al. 1979).

Total protein, total albumin and total globulin estimates are also taken. These reflect hepatic function (particularly albumin, which is made in the liver) as well as absorption and inflammation. Except in lupoid hepatitis, which can mimic rheumatoid arthritis, bilirubin and SGOT are likely to be normal.

NSAIDs may induce liver enzyme abnormalities, and it may be difficult to differentiate between drug effects and disease activity without discontinuation of NSAID therapy. NSAIDs seldom cause serious liver deterioration. Liver involvement may be present in up to 65% of patients with Felty's syndrome (Thorne et al. 1982).

Bone metabolism

Calcium, phosphate and alkaline phosphatase are all measured. Calcium is bound to protein and this may need a correction factor if protein levels are abnormal, as can occur in rheumatoid arthritis. A slightly raised calcium and raised alkaline phophatase level, if of bony origin, should alert the clinician to the possibility of osteomalacia. In Paget's disease there is a markedly raised alkaline phosphatase of bony origin. Radiographic confirmation of Paget's disease should be sought since secondary cancer in bone can also cause a raised alkaline phosphatase.

Renal function

Kidney involvement is usually sparse in rheumatoid arthritis, although a low grade nephropathy, glomerulitis vasculitis and secondary amyloidosis have all been described (Matteson et al. 1994). More commonly, renal abnormalities result from agents used in the treatment of rheumatoid arthritis, notably gold, D-Penicillamine, cyclosporin and the NSAIDs (Samuels et al. 1977). The renal involvement caused by nephrotoxic drugs is more likely to be seen first on routine urine testing.

Electrolytes (sodium, potassium, chloride and bicarbonate) together with urea and creatinine are usually measured. The chronic renal failure of connective tissue disorders may produce a raised potassium and a low bicarbonate level. The renal function in a normal subject will deteriorate throughout adult life. Urea may be raised because of dehydration but creatinine is less likely to do so under those circumstances. The creatinine is the most sensitive simple estimation of renal damage and a raised level may indicate amyloidosis or chronic renal failure.

Amyloidosis

Amyloidosis may develop in patients with rheumatoid arthritis as a result of long-standing active inflammation and cause proteinuria. It is not specific to the kidneys and may affect other organs including the heart, liver, spleen, intestines and skin. The diagnosis of

amyloidosis is confirmed by biopsy of the tissue involved. Unfortunately, the presence of secondary amyloidosis in patients with
rheumatoid arthritis heralds a poor outcome.

Assessment of rheumatic disease activity

Rheumatoid factor (RF)

Rheumatoid factor is a commonly requested immunlogical investigation. It is found in the blood of 75% of patients with rheumatoid
arthritis of more than 12 months duration but in only 40–50% of
those with early disease. The absence of rheumatoid factor therefore
does not preclude a diagnosis of rheumatoid arthritis; indeed, the
diagnosis of rheumatoid arthritis is not made on the presence of
rheumatoid factor alone but includes a host of other factors. If the
rheumatoid factor is absent and the patient has rheumatoid arthritis,
the arthritis is said to be *seronegative*.

Rheumatoid factor, an IgM/IgG complex of two immunoglobulins, can also be found in other conditions including liver disease,
sarcoidosis, subacute bacterial endocarditis, and in 4% of healthy
adults. It is detected by one or more of the following tests:

- sheep cell agglutination (Rose Waaler) test
- latex agglutination test
- RAHA test.

The result of the Rose Waaler test is given as a titre; below 1:32 is
not significant, 1:64 is positive and values above 1:500 usually indicate severe rheumatoid disease.

Antinuclear antibody (ANA)

The antinuclear antibody is regarded as an initial screening test for
systemic lupus erythematosus, but it is not specific for this condition
and if the result is positive the clinician will proceed to request DNA
binding from the same patient before confirming a diagnosis of
lupus. Antinuclear antibody can occur in other connective tissue
disorders such as systemic sclerosis, and occasionally in low titre in
rheumatoid arthritis. The titre is important, and values of 1 : 200 or
more in the presence of antiDNA antibodies are likely to confirm the
diagnosis of lupus.

Extractable nuclear antigen (ENA)

Testing extractable nuclear antigen is helpful for the diagnosis of mixed connective tissue disorder (Golding 1981).

Immunoglobulins

Immunoglobulin testing can provide useful information when the ESR is raised for no obvious reason. In seropositive rheumatoid arthritis serum IgM is usually though not always raised, representing rheumatoid factor in the blood. Equally, there may be a polyclonal increase of all immunoglobulins such as IgA, IgG and IgM.

IgA synthesised in mucous membranes may be raised in Sjogren's syndrome.

Plasma proteins and electrophoresis

The alpha z globulin is an acute phase reactant which when elevated indicates tissue destruction in the early phases of rheumatic disease. In the later stages a raised gammaglobulin may indicate antibody formation and very high levels can occur in connective tissue diseases, sarcoidosis and myelomatosis (Golding 1981).

Erythrocyte sedimentation rate (ESR)

The ESR is used as the standard test in many hospitals for evaluating disease activity in rheumatic disease. If inflammation is present in the body the ESR increases owing to the changes in the patient's blood. A quantity (2 ml) of anticoagulated blood is sucked in to a capillary tube and the speed with which red and white cells settle over a period of 1 hour is observed. Normal values vary with age and sex. ESR is of value in distinguishing inflammatory polyarthritis from the degenerative conditions.

ESR is elevated in rheumatoid arthritis, ankylosing spondylitis, acute gout, polymyalgia rheumatica, systemic connective tissue disorders, reactive and infective arthritis. A persistently raised ESR should alert the clinician to the possibility of myeloma (a malignant condition of the plasma cells). If suspected, urine should be collected to test for Bence Jones protein (a characteristic protein produced by the cell).

The ESR is not normally elevated in degenerative metabolic joint disease or in soft tissue rheumatism. The Westergren method of establishing the ESR is now universally used. ESRs of up to 20 mm/h in males and 25 mm/h in females are accepted as being within normal limits in rheumatological practice. (Golding 1981).

Plasma viscosity (PV)

The plasma viscosity test mimics ESR evaluation but studies the movement of the plasma in horizontal rather than vertical plane. Plasma viscosity eliminates the variation caused by the anaemia of rheumatoid arthritis which can influence the ESR. High values are found in active rheumatoid arthritis.

C-reactive protein (CRP)

C-reactive protein is an acute inflammatory protein produced by the liver in response to infections, inflammation or acute injury. It rises in active rheumatoid arthritis falling back to normal levels once the disease has come under control. Changes in the C-reactive protein occur faster than in other biochemical assessments. Levels remain normal in systemic lupus erythematosus.

Other acute phase reactants

Fibrinogen, hepatoglobin and *caeruloplasmin* all behave as acute phase reactants with high levels found in active disease and low values apparent as the conduction comes under control (Golding 1981).

Urine testing

Urinalysis, the examination of urine, is a valuable tool for the diagnosis and screening of several conditions. It also plays an important role in the surveillance of drug therapy, especially in terms of toxicity. This will be discussed in greater depth later in the chapter. A patient who is asked to supply a specimen of urine for testing requires the following:

- explanation of the reason for testing
- instruction in the method of collecting the specimen
- provision of suitable equipment, including a container for the specimen and washing facilities
- an appropriate environment including wherever possible visual and auditory privacy and adequate time (Cook 1996).

Appearance

The appearance of the urine should be noted for colour and clarity.

- Colour changes may be due to *endogenous pigments* such as *haemoglo-bin* (red/brown colour), *bilirubin* (yellow) or *intact red cells* (smoky red).
- *Exogenous pigments* may also cause colour changes, such as contamination with menstrual blood. The administration of sulphasalazine can cause orange discoloration.
- *Cloudiness* is caused by suspended particles which will settle on standing to leave a deposit. Normal urine may contain some renal tubular cells and a few white and red blood cells; these will be prevalent in certain diseases, contributing to a cloudy appearance (Cook 1996).

Odour

Normal; freshly voided urine has very little odour but will develop an ammoniacal smell if left for any length of time. Infected urine has a characteristic fishy smell. The urine of patients with anorexia, or a ketoacidosis diabetic person, has a sweet smell. The administration of sulphasalazine and/or D-Penicillamine can also cause a characteristic odour.

Specific gravity

Specific gravity of the urine can be measured using either reagent strips or a specially calibrated hydrometer. It indicates the ability of the kidneys to concentrate or dilute urine. A low specific gravity can occur if a patient has a high intake of fluid, or may indicate renal abnormalities or the presence of diabetes insipidus. A raised specific gravity may indicate dehydration.

Routine testing of urine may detect the following:

- *Glucose:* this is not usually found in urine. Its presence may be due to raised blood glucose levels or to reduced renal absorption. It can be associated with conditions such as diabetes mellitus, stress, cushing's syndrome and acute pancreatitis. Glycosuria occurring in the urine of a patient with rheumatic disease alerts the clinician to the possibility of corticosteroid induced diabetes mellitus.

- *Bilirubin;* in the urine may be indicative of hepatic or bilary disease. It may also be present if the patient has been prescribed phenothiazides or chlorpromazine, leading to a false positive result.
- *Ketones:* these are not normal constituents of urine. They are the produces of the breakdown of fatty acids, and their presence may indicate starvation, excessive dieting or uncontrolled diabetes (Cook 1996).
- *Blood:* often found to be of no significance, but should be investigated if persistent. It may be due to trauma, infection, tumour or stones. Haematuria is an early sign of polyarteritis and 50% of patients with lupus will have small amounts of blood and protein in their urine.
- *Protein;* can indicate a range of conditions including renal disease, urinary tract infection, hypertension, pre-eclampsia or congestive heart failure. Transient positive tests are not always significant and normal urine contains small amounts of albumin and globulin although not usually at a level that would be detected positively on a reagent strip. When testing for urinary protein, a morning specimen of urine is recommended to ensure sufficient concentration (Cook 1996). Proteinuria may be the first sign of a collagen disease such as polyarteritis. In rheumatoid disease it may indicate urinary infections, nephropathy due to gold or D-Penicillamine, or be secondary to amyloid diseases. If proteinuria persists, a 24-hour urine specimen should be requested; more than 0.15 g protein/24 hours is abnormal; over 1 g/24 hours is found when there is renal tubular damage, and in nephrosis well over 5 g protein/24 hours can occur (Golding 1981). The presence of albuminuria on routine testing often indicates a simple infection that will require treatment to prevent aggravation of a flare of rheumatoid arthritis, but it may also indicate glomerular dysfunction in conditions such as lupus.
- *Urobilinogen:* found normally in urine but increased levels may indicate liver abnormalities or excessive destruction of red blood cells such as in haemolytic anaemia (Cook 1996).
- *Nitrate:* not normally present in urine. It is produced when gram negative bacteria such as *Escherichia coli* convert dietary nitrates (e.g. from the preservative in meat products and cheese and in smoked foods) to nitrites. As *E. coli* is responsible for 80% of urine infections (Talaro and Talaro 1993), the presence of nitrites is strongly suggestive of urinary tract infection. The specimen for

testing should have been in the bladder for at least 4 hours before voiding to allow sufficient time for the nitrate/nitrite conversion.

- *Leukocytes:* the presence of leukocytes in the urine is an indication of bladder or renal infection, but follow-up testing such as urine culture is required. White blood cells should be sought in the urine when infections such as Reiter's disease are suspected. Early morning specimens are more likely to contain tubercule bacilli than those taken later in the day if the condition is suspected.

Record keeping

The results of the urinalysis should be recorded in the patient's records as soon as possible after testing. The United Kingdom Central Council's standards for records and record keeping (UKCC 1993) state that failure to keep accurate documentation neglects patients' interest by 'failing to focus attention on early signs of deviation from the norm and failing to place on record significant observations and conclusion'. It is worth noting that a negative result on a particular date may acquire significance in retrospect, so all results should be recorded in patients' records at the time of testing (Cook 1996).

3.4 When surveillance is required

SODIUM AUROTHIOMALATE (MYOCRISIN)

Treatment regime

Gold is used as long-term treatment for inflammatory joint disease (most commonly rheumatoid arthritis). Initially most patients are given an test dose of 10 mg intramuscularly, and if no adverse effects are experienced progress to 50 mg intramuscularly weekly, reducing to 50 mg fortnightly as the patient responds, normally around 6 months. With adequate control, frequency is reduced to monthly (around 12 months) and continued indefinitely until side effects occur.

It may take 3–6 months for patients to respond to treatment with gold. There are vast variations in the implementation of gold therapy. Kay and Puller (1992) found that in a survey of 100 rheumatologists 89% used a test dose of intramuscular gold, but of those who gave a test dose 64% gave a single 10 mg dose, 9% gave 10 mg followed by 20 mg, 4.5% gave 5 mg followed by 10 mg and the remaining rheumatologists gave various slowly increasing incremental doses. As stated earlier, the nurse will need to be familiar with the data sheet recommendations even if the unit policy differs from them. In the establishment of protocols it may well be worth noting that the data sheet recommendations were considered when establishing new policies for drug surveillance.

Adverse effects

Toxicity with injectible gold is common, occurring in 30–40% of patients (Day 1994).

Nephrotoxicity

It is the responsibility of the nurse administering the intramuscular injection of gold to test the urine prior to giving the injection. Minor transient proteinuria is common when a patient is on this therapy. A meta-analysis of clinical trials showed significant proteinuia in patients receiving gold (Day 1994). A trace of proteinuia can be ignored but increasing proteinuria is an indication to stop gold. Treatment should be discontinued if 24-hour protein urinalysis exceeds 1 g. Recovery is usual when gold is stopped.

Minor renal effects in the absence of proteinuria have been noted, with the elevation of enzymes and tubular cell secretion, but this increased turnover of tubular cells has not been related to decreased tubular function later in life (Ganley et al. 1989). Isolated microscopic haematuria is not usually attributed to gold (Leonard et al. 1987).

Muscocutaneous reactions

Dermatitis and *oral reactions* account for 60–80% of all reactions to injectible gold complexes (Champion et al. 1990). Oral mucosal lesions occur less often than rashes. Minor ulcers can be treated symptomatically. Check that ill-fitting dentures are not causing friction. Most rashes are usually erythematous and macular but rarely can exfoliate; 85% of rashes are severely pruritic.

Raised eosinophils may be the forerunner to a rash, and the rash may be associated with a metallic taste and organ toxicity such as proteinuria (Champion et al. 1990). Minor rashes and/or pruritis can be treated symptomatically with aqueous cream or 0.5 % hydro-cortisone cream.

The nurse should also establish that the cause of the rash is related to drug therapy, so that the treatment is not discontinued unnecessarily. This means checking that patients have not recently changed their soap or washing powder, or commenced new drug therapy. In some units close co-operation with the dermatologist can establish the cause of the rash and/or irritation and thus may provide valuable information in planning longterm care.

Gold should be withheld if there is a widespread pruritis, severe or rapidly progressive rash and/or mouths ulcers/stomatitis as these can be associated with exfoliative dermatitis. Once a moderate rash and/or pruritis has settled it may be possible to reintroduce gold at a smaller dose.

Haematological disorders

- *Neutropenia.* It is important to consider whether a decrease in white blood cells is due to the disease or related condition (e.g. Felty's syndrome) or to the gold treatment. Careful attention needs to be paid to a rapid and/or progressive downward trend in neutrophils accompanied by a fall in platelets, as this is often caused by bone marrow suppression as a direct result of gold treatment. (It is worth noting that you can also get neutropenia related to gold without an accompanying fall of other blood cells.) Increasing neutropenia will require increased surveillance, possible dosage reduction or cessation of gold.
- *Eosinophilia* will occur in up to 50% of patients receiving gold at some stage of their treatment and, although it does not generally correlate highly with toxicity, it should not be dismissed as in some cases it may herald a toxic reaction to treatment (Elderman et al. 1983).
- *Thrombocytopenia* occurs in 1–3% of patients receiving intra muscular gold. It is usually minor but can be serious (Day 1994). It usually responds well to corticosteroids.
- *Aplastic anaemia* is rare but has a high mortality rate, although the rate for survival is improving (Yan and Davies 1990).

Pulmonary involvement

- *Inflammation lung reactions: hypersensitivity pneumoconitis,* distinguishable from rheumatoid lung by its acute or subacute onset, can occur and will necessitate cessation of gold. *Obliterative bronchiolitis* has been reported in patients with rheumatoid arthritis but it remains unclear whether this is a result of gold therapy or the condition itself.
- Pulmonary involvement in patients with rheumatoid arthritis is fairly common, although the clinical features may be subtle (Matteson et al. 1994). *Pleurisy* and *pleural effusions* may improve spontaneously or require treatment. The occurrence of persistent pleural effusions will lead to fibrosis.
- Seropositive rheumatoid arthritis patients may develop *parenchymal pulmonary nodules* which, although usually asymptomatic, can cause pleural effusions.
- *Caplan's syndrome (pneumoconiosis)* is characterised by large multiple pulmonary nodules and is seen in individuals who have experienced prolonged exposure to coal dust.

- *Isolated pulmonary arteritis* is a rare complication of rheumatoid arthritis and is frequently associated with interstitial fibrosis and nodulosis.

Neurotoxicity

Neurotoxic reactions are uncommon but diverse reactions have been noted, including peripheral neuropathy, Guillain–Barré syndrome, cranial nerve palsies and encephalopathy.

Vasomotor reactions

Vasomotor reactions may occur within minutes of administration of the gold injection, necessitating that the patient remains in clinic for a period of time following the injection, These are often referred to as 'nitroid' reactions and are characterised by weakness, dizziness, nausea, sweating, facial flushing, erythema and hypotension.

Postinjection reactions

Apart from the possibility of vasomotor reactions, the patient may also experience transient polyarthralgia, myalgia, joint swelling, fatigue and malaise. It can be difficult at times to distinguish these effects from the symptoms of active inflammatory disease.

Incidence rate of side effects

A meta-analysis of clinical trials (Clarke et al. 1989) found that 11% of all patients had to discontinue gold because of side effects experienced. The majority of side effects occurs within the first 12 months of treatment and their occurrence is not related to cumulative dose (Sambrook et al. 1982). Lockie and Smith (1988), reporting their experience with gold therapy in 1019 patients, found the main reasons for discontinuation of gold to be skin reactions in 36% of patients and buccal irritation in 13%.

Reasons for stopping treatment

Gold should be stopped if:

- total white cell count is $<3 \times 10^9/L$ or neutrophils $<2 \times 10^9/L$
- platelets $<120 \times 10^9/L$
- proteinuria >1 g/24 hours
- there is a severe or progressive rash.

The majority of adverse reactions to gold resolve spontaneously within weeks to months following cessation of treatment.

AURANOFIN (RIDAURA)

Treatment regime

Auranofin is used in the long term treatment of rheumatoid arthritis. The usual dose is 3 mg twice daily. The absorption of gold from auranofin following a single dose is about 20–25%, and there is less retention of gold in tissues than occurs with injectible gold. Nevertheless regular blood monitoring is required.

Adverse effects

- *Rashes:* minor rashes can be treated symptomatically (aqueous cream, 0.5% hydrocortisone cream).
- *Mouth ulcers:* minor ulcers can be treated with Bonjela, Difflam mouth wash or Adcortyl in orabase.
- *Gastrointestinal problems:* diarrhoea is often the commonest side effect and may respond to the introduction of bulking agents such as bran or to a temporary reduction in dosage. Some patients experience nausea and vomiting, and it is recommend that this therapy is taken with food.
- *Renal problems:* proteinuria.
- *Haematological problems:* the nurse must observe for any reductions in neutrophils and platelets.
- *Miscellaneous:* rarely colitis, peripheral neuritis, pulmonary fibrosis, hepatotoxicity with cholestatic jaundice and alopecia have all been reported.

Reasons for stopping treatment

Auranofin should be stopped if:

1. total white cell count is $<3 \times 10^9/L$
2. platelets $<120 \times 10^9/L$
3. proteinuria >1 g/24 hours
4. severe rashes or severe mouth ulcers occur.

D-PENICILLAMINE (DISTAMINE)

Treatment regime

D-Penicillamine is used in the long term treatment of rheumatoid arthritis and in scleroderma. Treatment is commenced at 125 mgs or 250 mg daily, increasing at 4 week intervals by increments of 125 mg daily to 500 mg or 750 mg. The tablets are best taken as a single daily dose an hour before breakfast and not with iron tablets or milk as they interfere with drug absorption. Toxicity is common with this treatment, with about 50% of patients with rheumatoid arthritis experiencing an adverse effect within the first 6 months of treatment at 600 mg daily resulting in 25% of patients discontinuing with this treatment. The incidence of toxicity increases as the dose increases (Kay 1986).

Adverse reactions

Mucocutaneous reactions

Urticarial, pruritic, macular, papular eruptions of apparent allergic origin account for the majority of skin reactions (Kay 1986). Minor rashes can be treated symptomatically but severe rashes may necessitate stopping D-Penicillamine, which will normally resolve the rash. Autoimmune billous skin eruptions, typical of the pemphigus group, are the most worrying. Patients who have a penicillin allergy are at greater risk of experiencing a mucocutaneous reaction. Oral ulcers and stomatitis may occur; if they are severe this will mean a discontinuation of therapy. Oral mucosal involvement is often present in pemphigus. There is a significant level of mortality amongst patients with D-Penicillamine induced pemphigus. (Joyce 1990).

Taste

A metallic taste and loss of taste may occur in the first 8 weeks of treatment, and the patient may take several months to recover from it. This can be a particularly distressing symptom for patients, and advice may need to be given on food supplementation (Ryan 1995). Taste disturbance may be a consequence of zinc chelation by the D-Penicillamine, but zinc therapy does not remove the complaint (Joyce 1990).

Nausea and anorexia

If these symptoms occur the patient may need to reduce the dose of D-Penicillamine and then increase slowly when the symptoms settle. The use of antiemetics should also be considered.

Haematological effects

There can be a gradual or rapid haematological effects at any stage during treatment with D-Penicillamine. Thromobocytopenia can occur. Neutropenia due to D-Penicillamine as opposed to rheumatoid arthritis itself is suggested by a rapid or progressive fall in neutrophils and is the commonest cause of death attributed to this treatment (Kay 1979). Aplastic anaemia also has a high fatality rate.

Renal involvement

Proteinuria is common. Increased urinary protein excretion can exceed 0.5 g/day in approximately 9% of patients taking this drug (Stein et al. 1986). The presence of HLA-B8 and HLA-DR4 antigens, coupled with the occurrence of previous proteinuria on gold therapy, increases the risk of more severe proteinuria leading to nephrotic syndrome (Joyce 1990).

The majority of patients experiencing severe proteinuria have membranous glomerulonephritis with minimal change neuropathy. Plasma urea and creatinine may rise intermittently but this does not seem to be related to permanent renal impairment.

D-Penicillamine should be stopped if over 1 g of proteinuria occurs in a 24-hour period. Even after the drug has been discontinued the proteinuria may persist for up to 21 months.

The appearance of haematuria may indicate rapidly progressive glomerulonephritis, e.g. Goodpasture's syndrome or systemic lupuss erythematosus, and can be life threatening requiring steroids and immunosuppressives. However, the presence of haematuria usually does not lead to serious complication and recurrent haematuria is quite common in rheumatoid arthritis patients without serious renal pathology (Leonard et al. 1987).

Pulmonary involvement

Cases of *bronchiolitis obliterans* have been reported (Day 1994). Although this is a rare side effect it may be irreversible and present as dyspnoea late in therapy (Kay 1986).

Autoimmune reactions

Myasthenia gravis is a rare complication which may evolve after years of uneventful therapy and may take over a year to resolve (Kay 1986).

Autoantibodies may appear, including antistriated muscle antibody, anticentromere antibody and antiglomerular basement membrane antibody. The latter is associated with the life-threatening complication of Goodpasture's syndrome.

Dermatomyositis / polymyositis

Drug induced *systemic lupus erythematosus* usually resolves after stopping D-Penicillamine. *Pemphigus* (oral involvement common) is dangerous and requires cessation of D-Penicillamine, glucocorticosteroids and perhaps plasmapheresis.

Reasons for stopping treatment

D-Penicillamine should be stopped if:

- there is a severe rash or severe mouth ulcers.
- an autoimmune side effect occurs
- platelets $<120 \times 10^9/L$
- total white cell count $<3 \times 10^9/L$
- neutrophils $<2 \times 10^9/L$
- proteinuria >1 g/24 hours.

SULPHASALAZINE (SALAZOPYRIN)

Treatment regime

Sulphasalazine is used in its enteric coated form (EN) as second-line treatment for rheumatoid arthritis, spondyloarthropathies and reactive arthritis. To reduce nausea the drug should be commenced at 500 mg daily increasing by 500 mg daily at weekly intervals to the usual maintenance dose of 1 g twice daily. Incomplete responders sometimes require 1 gram three times a day. It may take 3–6 months for a patient to respond to treatment with sulphasalazine. This preparation ranks with the antimalarials and auranofin as the best tolerated of the DMARDs, and is the most popular first choice of DMARDs amongst rheumatologists (Kay and Puller 1992).

Adverse effects

These are commonest in the first 3 months of therapy. Only 20–25% of patients need to stop treatment because of toxicity and only about 5% of patients will experience potentially serious side effects (Farr et al. 1986).

Gastrointestinal and central nervous system involvement

Symptoms may include nausea, vomiting, malaise, anorexia, abdominal pain, dyspepsia, indigestion, headache, light headiness and dizziness.

- If a patient experiences *nausea* the dose should be reduced to the previously tolerated dose and further increase should be attempted slowly. Make sure the patient is taking enteric coated tablets and administering them on a full stomach. Antiemetics may be required.
- In the case of *headaches*, again the dose should be initially reduced and further increases attempted slowly. If headaches are severe the patient may need to discontinue sulphasalazine.
- *Pyrexia* is a rare side effect and can only be considered when other causes of raised temperature have been excluded.

Hypersensitivity

Hypersensitivity is relatively common and may manifest itself in a number of ways ranging from skin rash to fatal multiorgan involvement.

Skin

If there is a *mild rash*, treatment can be continued and the rash can be treated symptomatically. Skin rashes will occur within 5% of cases and take the form of a generalised pruritic maculopapular rash, urticaria or photosensitivity. If the rash occurs within the first 2 weeks of treatment then desensitisation can be tried. Initially given in 1 mg doses, sulphasalazine is built up over 25–56 days. Successful desensitisation has been achieved in as many as 85% of cases in rheumatoid arthritis patients (Bax and Amos 1986).

Rarely, severe reactions such as *Stevens–Johnson syndrome* or *exfoliative dermatitis* can occur. If this happens, all drugs should be stopped and urgent dermatological advice should be obtained. Rarely, *serum sickness* occurs.

Pulmonary involvement

Most toxicity is allergic in origin from sulphasalazine. The commonest presentation is eosinophilic pneumonitis; symptoms include dyspnoea with fever, rash, weight loss, pulmonary infiltration on radiograph and reduced pulmonary function tests. Reduction of symptoms occurs after cessation of therapy (Tydd and Dyer 1976).

Haematological effects

- *Leucopenia* occurs in 1–5 % of cases. It is most likely to occur in the first 6 months of treatment, although it can occur at any time. It is the commonest potential serious side effect associated with sulphasalazine. It indicates the need for continued review, particularly as early recognition with dosage reduction or cessation leads to reversal in most cases.
- *Thrombocytopenia* is less frequent than leucopenia.
- *Agranulocytosis* is rare but can develop rapidly and present with intercurrent infection. It has been recorded in association with a transient but marked plasmocytosis.
- Sulphasalazine causes the *erythrocyte mean cell volume (MCV)* to rise. It inhibits *folate* uptake in the small bowel; however, it would be rare to see folate deficiency at a dose of 2 g daily.
- *Abnormalities of red cell morphology* are due to oxidant damage resulting in red cell membrane abnormalities leading to low grade haemolysis (Pounder et al. 1973). The changes are reversible on discontinuation of therapy, but this action is necessary only if the haemolysis is causing a problem. Significant methaemoglobin can cause headaches and may require a dosage reduction.

Hepatoxicity

- *Allergic hepatic responses* to sulphonamides are well known; raised hepatic enzyme levels and eosinophilia may cause fever rash and hepatomegaly.
- *Granulomatous hepatitis* may occur, necessitating discontinuation of therapy. Minor rises in hepatic enzyme levels during treatment occur in about 3% of cases but do not seem to be productive of severe hepatic reactions, and treatment may continue (Puller et al. 1987).

- Liver function tests need to be carried out weekly for the first month and monthly thereafter for 6 months. It is then usual to check the liver function twice yearly.

Reversible oligospermia

Sulphasalazine should be avoided in men wishing to have a family, as 70% of men taking it develop oligospermia and abnormal sperm motility (Birnie et al 1981). This temporary reduction in fertility is reversible on stopping sulphasalazine treatment.

Miscellaneous

Sulphasalazine can cause orange staining of soft contact lenses. The urine can become bright orange. Rarely, drug induced lupus.

Reasons for stopping treatment

Sulphasalazine should be stopped if:

- severe rashes or severe headaches occur
- liver function deteriorates
- platelets <120 $\times$ 10^9/L
- total white cell count <3 $\times$ 10^9/L
- neutrophils <2 $\times$ 10^9/L.

METHOTREXATE

Treatment regime

Methotrexate is an antimetabolite cytotoxic agent used in rheumatoid arthritis, psoriatic arthritis, myositis and vasculitis. It is given weekly either orally or intramuscularly in doses between 5 mg and 25 mg per week. It is sometimes co-prescribed with folic acid, which reduces the likelihood of minor side effects. Clinical effect is usually evident after 2–3 months but doses may need to be increased to maintain this effect. A chest radiograph is taken prior to starting treatment, as pre-existing lung disease requires special attention. Alcohol should ideally be avoided. Trimethoprim and trimoxazole (Bactrim, Septrin) and phenytoin should not be prescribed in patients taking methotrexate because of their antifolate action.

Adverse effects

Gastrointestinal symptoms

These are the most common side effects, including anorexia, nausea, dyspepsia, vomiting, diarrhoea and abdominal pain. Antiemetics may be required on the day of methotrexate administration and the following 24–48 hours. If nausea and vomiting are a problem and there is doubt about absorption, methotrexate can be given intramuscularly.

Mouth ulcers

Mouth soreness can present with or without ulceration (Kremer and Joong 1986). The use of folic acid to minimise stomatitis has been recommended (Segal et al. 1990). Minor ulcers can be treated symptomatically but major mouth ulcers may necessitate dose reduction or discontinuation.

Rashes

Minor rashes can be treated symptomatically but severe rashes may necessitate discontinuation of methotrexate.

Haematological effects

Leucopenia is the most common bone marrow toxicity from methotrexate (Kremer and Joong 1986). This is usually managed by reducing the dosage of methotrexate. *Anaemia* and *thrombocytopenia* can also occur. *Macrocytosis* is a sign of toxicity and may precede bone marrow suppression.

Hepatoxicity

Hepatoxicity, defined as elevation of transaminase, occurs in 69–89% of patients. These increases do not usually correlate with the development of cirrhosis. The consensus appears to be that a pretreatment liver biopsy is not usually necessary unless risk factors such as previous alcoholism exist, although there is still debate that periodic liver biopsies may be required after commencement of treatment (Segal et al. 1990). Acute hepatitis and reversible hepatic failure has been reported (Clegg et al. 1989). The practitioner should consider stopping treatment if there is a persistent elevation of AST or ALT. Liver function should be assessed biochemically weekly for the first month and monthly thereafter.

Hypersensitivity reactions and pneumonitis

Hypersensitivity reactions include rashes, fever and pneumonitis (Cannon et al. 1983). Acute pneumonitis is potentially serious and should be considered if there is a dry cough and recent breathlessness.

Pulmonary hypersensitivity with severe hypoxia seems to occur in 2–6% of patients and is not dose related but associated with eosinophilia (Alarcon et al. 1989). Recurrent pulmonary disease after treatment with methotrexate has been reported (Kaplan and Waite 1978).

Renal involvement

Acute renal decompensation and renal failure have been reported, although rarely, and appear related to high dose therapy with concomitant NSAIDs with underlying renal disease (Thierry et al. 1989). Renal function should be assessed biochemically weekly for the first month and then monthly thereafter.

Infections

There is an ongoing debate that patients recovering methotrexate are at increased risk of herpes zoster (Wilke and Mackenzie 1986).

Reasons for stopping treatment

Methotrexate should be stopped if:

- major mouth ulcers or severe skin rashes occur
- acute pneumonitis occurs
- liver function deteriorates
- platelets $<120 \times 10^9$/L
- total white blood cell count $<3 \times 10^9$/L
- neutrophils $<2 \times 10^9$/L.

AZATHIOPRINE (IMURAN)

Treatment regime

Azathioprine is an immunosuppressant antimetabolite used in

rheumatoid arthritis, psoriatic arthritis and vasculitis. It is widely used to suppress transplant rejection. It is given orally in daily doses of up to 2.5 mg/kg. It can be used in combination with corticosteroids as a 'steroid sparing agent'. It may take 3–6 months for patients to respond to treatment.

Adverse effects

Gastrointestinal symptoms

Intolerance to azathioprine can occur (Zarday et al. 1972). This includes *nausea and vomiting*. Patients may have to reduce the dose and then increase it again when symptoms settle. Antiemetics may be required. It is advisable to take azathioprine on a full stomach.

Mouth ulcers

Minor ulcers can be treated symptomatically but severe ulceration may necessitate stopping azathioprine.

Hepatoxicity

This is rare, but if occurs it may be severe and require dose reduction or withdrawal. Liver function tests should be carried out weekly for the first month of treatment and then monthly thereafter.

Haematological effects

The most important side effect is *reversible marrow suppression* (Luqmani et al. 1990). A full blood count is required weekly for the first month of treatment and then monthly thereafter. *Macrocytosis* is common but is not a sign of toxicity.

Lymphoma

Long-term effects may include the induction of lymphoid tumours (Rossman and Bertino 1973). In rheumatoid arthritis the azathioprine related risk of lymphoma and non-Hodgkin's lymphoma is confounded by an increased relative risk secondary to rheumatoid arthritis. Overall there appears to be a small added risk of developing malignancy when using azathioprine in rheumatoid arthritis (Furst and Clements 1994).

Miscellaneous

Hypersensitive reactions occur early in treatment and may include headaches, confusion and aseptic meningitis.

Drug interactions

Allopurinol can increase the myelosuppression of azathioprine.

Reason for stopping therapy

Azathioprine should be stopped if:

- platelets $<120 \times 10^9/L$
- white cell count $<3 \times 10^9/L$
- neutrophils $<2 \times 10^9/L$
- liver function deteriorates.

CYCLOPHOSPHAMIDE (ENDOXANA)

Treatment regime

Cyclophosphamide is a cytotoxic alleylating agent used for immuno-suppression in systemic lupus erythematosus, vasculitis, resistant rheumatic arthritis , polyarteritis nodosa, Wegener's granulomatosis, myositis and as a steroid sparing agent. A daily oral dose of 1–2 mg/kg body weight is used; it may be given as pulsed intravenous or oral therapy.

Cyclophosphamide reaches its peak of effectiveness after approximately 16 weeks, and although remission may be maintained for several years on withdrawal of the drug the majority of patients will experience some recurrence of symptoms. Non-articular complications of rheumatoid arthritis such as interstitial lung disease, cutaneous ulcers and peripheral neuropathy may respond well to oral cyclophosphamide. Cyclophosphamide should be used with care in patients with diabetes as it may induce hyper- or hypoglycaemia.

Pretreatment check

- Avoid cyclophosphamide if possible in men and women of child bearing age. Otherwise offer gamete storage and ensure adequate contraception.

- Carry out a full infection screen including chest, urine testing and culture, joint examination, sinuses and perineum.
- Some rheumatology units advise patients on this therapy to minimise or stop alcohol consumption.
- Pretreatment investigations include chest radiograph and a full blood count, including differential white count and platelets, electrolytes and liver function tests.

Adverse effects

Mouth ulcers

Minor ulcers can be treated symptomatically. Severe ulcers may necessitate stopping cyclophosphamide.

Nausea and vomiting

If gastrointestinal intolerance occurs the patient may require antiemetic therapy. It is advisable to take this treatment with food.

Alopecia

This is usually mild in dosages less than 100 mg daily.

Infections

Suppression of the immune system exposes patients to the risk of infections. This can be minor, e.g. herpes zoster, or major, e.g. septicaemia. There is also an increased risk of patients experiencing opportunistic infections.

Haemorrhagic cystitis

Bladder toxicity is due mainly to the effects of acrolein on the urinary metabolite of cyclophosphamide. As well as causing haemorrhagic cystitis and bladder fibrosis, it has been associated with bladder carcinoma, so the occurrence of haemorrhagic cystitis is an indication for cessation of therapy. Haemorrhagic cystitis has been reported in about a third of subjects receiving oral cyclophosphamide daily (Baker et al. 1987). It is rare in patients receiving intermittent high dose intravenous cyclophosphamide therapy (Bacon 1987), where it is often co-prescribed with mesna which reacts specifically with the metabolite acrolein preventing urothelial toxicity. Patients should be advised to take at least 3 litres of fluid per day while taking cyclophosphamide therapy.

Malignancy

Kinlen et al. (1979) reports a relative risk of 12.8 for all cancers combined and a 10-fold increase in bladder cancer for patients receiving at least 3 months of treatment with cyclophosphamide. There appear to be a relationship between total dose and duration of therapy and the incidence of malignancy (Baker et al. 1987). There is also an increased risk of leukaemia (Adamson and Seiber 1981).

Fertility

The risk of infertility, azoosperma and amenorrhoea with cyclophosphamide increases with higher dosages, longer duration of therapy and increased age in women (Schilsky et al. 1980). Infertility is not always reversible.

Pulmonary fibrosis

This can occur with therapy.

Haematological effects

Abnormalities are detected by blood monitoring. A full blood count is obtained weekly for the first month of treatment and then monthly thereafter. Maximum effect on the marrow dose not occur until 5–10 days after dosage. Recovery is seen within 10–14 days. *Macrocytosis* is not inevitable but is a sign of toxicity and dosage reduction may be necessary.

Drug interactions

Allopurinol can increase the myelosuppression of cyclophosphamide.

Reasons for stopping treatment

Cyclophosphamide should be stopped if:

- severe mouth ulcers occur
- platelets $<120 \times 10^9/L$
- total white cell count $<3 \times 10^9/L$
- neutrophils $<2 \times 10^9/L$
- there is macroscopic haematuria or persistent confirmed macroscopic haematuria (infection excluded).

Cyclosporin

Treatment regime

Cyclosporin A is a fungal metabolite of *Trichoderma polysporum* and *Cyclocarpon leucidium*. Studies have confirmed the potent effects of this drug in several arthritic and other cell mediated chronic inflammatory conditions (Cannon et al. 1990). Cyclosporin therapy may be instituted after a discussion of the risks (particularly nephrotoxicity), definition of treatment goals, clinical history, physical examination and laboratory testing. It may be instituted at doses of 2.5 mg/kg per day, given in two divided doses every 12 hours. The dose may be cautiously increased 25–50% every 2–4 weeks until a maximum of 5 mg/kg per day is reached, assuming there are no adverse reactions. Cyclosporin is used in the treatment of rheumatoid arthritis and Behcet's disease. Clinical improvements in patients receiving cyclosporin are associated with a reduction in C-reactive protein, d-1-acidglycoprotein and platelet counts, but not rheumatoid factor or ESR. (Dougados et al. 1988). When cyclosporin is used in the treatment of rheumatic disease, side effects are generally mild and reversible at low doses (Furst and Clements 1994).

Adverse effects

Minor reactions can include *nausea and vomiting, tinnitus, tremor, paraesthesia* and *gum hyperplasia*.

NEPHROTOXICITY

Cyclosporin should be avoided in patients with pre-existing renal disease. Increases in serum creatinine are common during cyclosporin immunosuppression. Cyclosporin therapy in doses of 10 mg/kg per day for even 2 months may lead to an irreversible loss of more than 10% of renal function in rheumatoid arthritis patients. Nephrotoxicity is dose related (Berg et al. 1989). Long-term influences on renal function are significant even after cessation of the drug, especially in view of the potential for apparent persistent impairment of creatinine clearance. Although a study by Tugwell et al. (1990) showed that although serum creatinine rose and creatinine clearance decreased over the period of cyclosporin administration, the effects stabilised after 4 months with no further changes. After discontinuation of therapy, serum creatinine fell to within 15% of baseline in all except two patients. Dosage reductions of 25–50% are required if serum creatinine increases above baseline by 30–50% or if hypertension cannot be controlled. Weekly serum creatinine measurements are required as long as the cyclosporin dose is being adjusted. Once the cyclosporin dose is stable, a serum creatinine measurement every 2–4 weeks should be adequate. Tests for cyclosporin levels are possible but the levels obtained do not clearly reflect cyclosporin toxicity efficacy. If these levels are monitored trough values >300 mg/ml should be avoided (Kowal et al. 1990).

Hypertension

Hypertension has always been a factor predisposing to nephrotoxicity in rheumatoid arthritis (Shiroky et al. 1989). New onset hypertension has been reported in about one third of rheumatoid arthritis and psoriatic patients. Hypertension should be managed with beta blockers and ACE inhibitors. Potassium-sparing diuretics should be avoided because cyclosporin may cause hyperkalemia (Kowal at al 1990).

Hepatoxicity

This can occur with higher dosages of cyclosporin and present with elevated hepatic enzymes and bilirubin.

Drug interactions

Diltiazem, ketaconazole, rifampicin and phenytoin may all require adjustment of cyclosporin dose.

Reasons for stopping treatment

Cyclosporin should be discontinued if:

• elevation of serum creatinine persists even after dosage reduction
• there is uncontrollable hypertension
• cyclosporin levels are >300 mg/ml
• hepatic enzymes are elevated.

Chlorambucil

Treatment regime

Chlorambucil, like cyclophosphamide, is a bifunctional alkylating agent. It is not cytotoxic but is metabolised to phenylacetic acid its principal and most active metabolite. It is given in an oral preparation. The intravenous preparation is unstable because of rapid hydrolysis. Chlorambucil can be commenced in doses of 0.1–0.2 mg/kg per day. Once response or toxicity has occurred it is suggested that a dose between 3 and 4 mg daily is adopted.

Chlorambucil has been used in patients with rheumatoid arthritis, vasculitis and connective tissue disorders, inflammatory eye disease and amyloidosis.

Adverse effects

The advantages of chlorambucil therapy have to be balanced against the risk of inducing adverse effects. The most common toxicities with chlorambucil use are dose-related bone marrow suppression and infertility.

Bone marrow suppression

Cumulative bone marrow toxicity occurs regularly and often required discontinuation of the drug.

Neoplasms

Kahn et al. (1979) reported that leukaemias occurred in patients with rheumatoid arthritis who had received a total dose of at least 1 g of chlorambucil and who had been treated for at least 6 months. Luqmani et al. (1990), reviewing the literature on patients receiving chlorambucil, indicated that tumours occurred in less than 1% of patients. The majority of the malignancies were leukaemias, with a particularly high incidence of acute myeloid leukaemia. It is not possible to exclude the part that the disease process itself plays in the likelihood of malignancies, and Palmer and Denman (1984) found that patients with connective tissue disorders were more sensitive to the leukaemiogenic effects of chlorambucil than patients with other non-malignant conditions.

Infertility

The risk of infertility, azoospermia and amenorrhoea increase with duration of therapy and high doses. Infertility effects men at a greater rate than women. Irreversible azospermia was regularly reported in men receiving more than 400 mg of chlorambucil. In postpubertal females both gametogenesis and hormonal function are altered adversely and menopause occurs.

PHENYLBUTAZONE (BUTACOTE)

Treatment regime

Phenylbutazone is no longer recommended or indeed available in many countries for the treatment of arthritis conditions, owing to the risk of marrow aplasia. Although it is still used in this country, it is available only on hospital prescription for patients with ankylosing spondylitis and other spondyloarthropathies. Phenylbutazone is a NSAID but it may also effect the immune response (Furst 1988). It is usually prescribed in dosages of 100–200 mg, 2–3 times a day. It should help with pain and swelling within a week but will take months before an immune response can be assessed.

Adverse effects

- *Gastrointestinal:* nausea and vomiting.
- *Mucocutaneous:* skin rashes, mouth ulcers, stomatitis.
- *Central nervous system:* headaches, dizziness and blurred vision.
- *Pulmonary toxicity:* care must be taken when prescribing these tablets to patients with asthma or breathing problems as these conditions may be aggravated.
- *Cardiovascular:* phenylbutazone has fluid retaining properties.
- *Hepatic:* serious hepatocellular reactions have been reported and hepatic clearance of drugs is reduced as phenylbutazone inhibits oxidaine drug metabolism.
- *Haematological abnormalities:* a range of haematological abnormalities have been reported. Long-term recipients may develop *iron deficiency anaemia* owing to chronic blood loss from inflammation of the small intestine. *Aplastic anaemia* has been associated with the slow metabolism of phenylbutazone (Leyland et al. 1974), suggesting that this adverse effect is related to excessive concentrations of the drug. *Thrombocytopenia*, effects on *platelet function, agranulocytosis, pancytopenia* and *haemolytic anaemia* have also been noted but are still rare although can be fatal (O'Brien and Bagly 1985).

Interactions

Phenylbutazone interacts with oral anticoagulants, lithium, oral hypoglycaemic agents, phenytoin, methotrexate, digoxin, aminoglycosides, probenecid and barbituates.

DAPSONE

Treatment regime

Dapsone is best known as an antileprotic agent but it also has effects on the immune system and has been used for the treatment of rheumatoid arthritis and psoriatic arthritis. There is a delay of 2–3 months before onset of action, but when successful it will reduce the ESR. The dosage is 50 mgs daily for 1 week then increasing to 100 mg daily depending on the result of the haemoglobin. Occasionally patients may require 150 mg daily.

Adverse effects

Minor side effects such as *rashes* and *gastric upset* can occur. Haematological effects include *haemolysis* which occurs in all patients and gives a drop in haemoglobin of 1–2 g. This therefore requires monitoring before increases in dosage are considered. Patients also develop a *pallor* which is more marked than the drop in the haemoglobin would imply. It is worth warning patients that they will look pale. Patients of Mediterranean origin will require a glucose 6-phosphatase dehydrogenase (G6PD) estimation prior to starting treatment since massive haemolysis will occur if there is a deficiency in this enzyme. *Agranulocytosis* has been reported but is rare.

MINOCYCLINE (MINOCIN)

Minocycline is a broad spectrum antibiotic often prescribed in the treatment of acne. It has also been used in the treatment of rheumatoid arthritis. Its mode of action is not known, but it is thought to be effective in inhibiting the proinflammatory enzyme metalloproteinase. It does not become fully effective for 2–3 months. The dosage is 100–300 mg twice daily.

Adverse effects

An abnormal *metallic taste* can occur when first starting the treatment. *Dizziness, nausea* and *diarrhoea* have also been reported. The treatment is best taken with food.

Although severe side effects are rare, a drug-induced lupus syndrome and hepatitis can occur that resolve on stopping but necessitate that treatment is monitored with a full blood count and biochemistry monthly and an antinuclear antibody 6 monthly.

Interactions

Minocycline should not be taken at the same time as antacids, calcium and iron preparations. A 2 hour gap is required between administration of minocycline and these preparations.

If prescribed penicillin, omit the minocycline until the course of penicillin is completed. Minocycline also interacts with warfarin.

Vaccination

Live vaccines (shown in Table 3.6) should be avoided in patients taking *azathioprine, methotrexate, cyclophosphamide* or high doses of corticosteroids. Patients on these medications should be considered for varicella-zoster immunoglobulin after exposure to chickenpox or herpes-zoster and should be advised to avoid close contact with patients recently vaccinated with live polio vaccine because of the risk of infections from fecal excretion.

Sulphasalazine, D-Penicillamine, gold – in general vaccination is safe for patients on these therapies, although it is probably preferable to avoid live vaccines.

Cyclosporin has a poor response to vaccines and patients should ideally have any appropriate vaccinations prior to therapy.

Pregnancy

Patients planning a family will require advice and support from various members of the rheumatology team. One of the major concerns of any pregnant woman is the risk of congenital malformation due to drugs, and this will cause even greater concern to the woman with rheumatoid arthritis (Richardson 1992). The most vulnerable period of gestation is during embryonic and fetal development, but many

Table 3.6 Vaccinations

Live vaccines	Inactivated vaccines
Measles	Influenza
Rubella	Typhoid (injected)
BCG	Poliomyelitis (IPV injected)
Mumps	Cholera
Poliomyelitis (OPV)	Diptheria
Yellow fever	Haemophilis influenza
Typhoid (oral)	Hepatitis A
	Hepatitis B
	Meningococcal
	Pertussis
	Pneumococcus
	Tetanus

congenital abnormalities occur for reasons other than those that are drug related. Spontaneous and serious malformations occur in 2–3 % of all pregnancies and minor malformation occur in a further 6% (Oka and Vainio 1966).

Woman with rheumatoid arthritis often need to achieve disease suppression to increase their chance of conceiving. Adequate control of the disease will enable a woman to feel capable of raising a child. Decisions regarding the withdrawal of potentially toxic drug therapy need to be made in good time, since many drugs can affect the vulnerable stages of embryogeniesis. Women should discontinue teratogenic agents such as methotrexate, azathioprine and cyclophosphamide at least 6 months before attempting conception. Ideally all drug therapy should be avoided during pregnancy and lactation (le Gallez 1988). The effects of drug therapy used in rheumatic disease are shown in Table 3.7.

In ankylosing spondylitis 80% of patients may experience a worsening of symptoms or no alteration of their condition during pregnancy (le Gallez 1988) and will require advice on coping with pain. This should include relaxation techniques, the application of hot and cold therapy and the use of diversional techniques. In rheumatoid arthritis 75% of women experience some remission of their condition during pregnancy but often return to disease status comparable with their prepregnant state within 8 months of giving birth. Women who develop an exacerbation of their condition postpartum will need to recommence their suppressive drug therapy and individual advice from the rheumatology nurse will be required if the mother is breast-feeding.

Table 3.7 Drugs and pregnancy

Drug	Effects if taken during pregnancy
Analgesics	
Paracetamol	can be taken during pregnancy
NSAIDs	May lead to the premature of the ductus gloriosus
Aspirin	Can cause cleft palate (in taken in first trimester) and antepartum haemorrhage
DMARDs	
Sulphasalazine	Neonatal jaundice
Antimalarials	Congenital blindness
Gold and D-Penicillamine	Not known
Cytotoxic medications	All teratogenic
Methotraxate	
Azathioprine	
Cyclophosphamide	
Corticosteroids	Can be taken in low dosages (<10 mg daily). If withdrawn prior to labour steroid cover will be required

Contraception

Reliable contraception should be advised for all women receiving DMARD therapy and all proposed pregnancies should be discussed on an individual basis with the rheumatology nurse. Patients (male and female) on medication known to be teratogenic, e.g. methotrexate, azathioprine and cyclophosphamide, must have contraceptive cover and discontinue the drug for 6 months before trying for a family.

Appendix: Drug monitoring clinic protocols

Reactions can occur in many sites. The nurse needs to be aware of:

- what to look for
- how to respond.

Skin manifestations

Changes in skin integrity can be related to:

- the disease process, i.e. vasculitis and leg ulcers
- the drugs used for therapy, i.e. gold injections
- difficulties faced in maintenance of skin integrity.

Rash

A rash

- may occur with any medication but is most commonly seen in those patients having gold therapy.
- can vary from minor eczematous lesions to severe widespread problem.

If a patient presents with a rash:

- Ask if they have recently changed their detergent. Consider sunburn, insect bites.
  - If the rash is isolated to an odd patch. Advise E45 cream. Review in a month's time.
  - If it is a severe, persistent or generalised rash, this may require a dermatology opinion – arrange referral.
- Sulphasalazine: if a rash occurs within the first 14 days commence desensitisation.

Itching

- troublesome itching – continue with treatment. Advise use of E45 cream or antihistamines. If the scalp is itchy, scaly or dry, advise a coal tar based solution, e.g. Baltar.
- Unbearable itching (i.e. cannot sleep because of it). Stop the medication and refer to the doctor's clinic.

Urinary manifestations

Urinary abnormalities may be due to:

- the disease itself (amyloid)
- gold or D-Penicillamine (less likely with sulphasalazine and methotrexate)
- asymptomatic urinary tract infections (which are common in rheumatoid arthritis patients)
- the ultrasensitivity of lab stick testing (i.e. false positives).

Proteinuria

- A trace or one + in isolation: ignore.
- ++ repeat dipstick testing, if ++ still present then send midstream specimen of urine (MSU). Patient and GP will be contacted if infection is present.
- If patient is symptomatic send MSU.
- If MSU reveals no infection but ++ persists, arrange 24-hour urine collection.
- When sending off an MSU, record on the form whether or not the patient is taking antibiotics.
- If +++ protein, stop treatment and collect 24-hour urine, unless the patient is known to have proteinuria.

Haematuria

- Confirm that the patient is not menstruating.
- A trace or one + in isolation: ignore.
- If ++ or +++ MSU – continue treatment.
- If the patient has observed blood loss: inform doctor.

Nitrate

- If nitrate positive with protein or blood – send MSU.
- Nitrate in isolation ignore.

Glycosuria

- If patient is a known diabetic – advise, refer back to diabetic monitoring.
- If not known to be diabetic arrange random blood sugar test. If over 11 mmol this is indicative of diabetes, and will require a fasting blood sugar test. Fasting blood sugar of over 8 mmol is indicative of diabetes.

Mouth

If the patient presents with a sore mouth:

- If dentures are worn, ensure these are fitted correctly.
- For minor ulcers (i.e. one or two in isolation) continue treatment. suggest Bonjela, Bioral Gel, Bioplex mouth rinse.
- For major mouth ulcers, i.e. acute severe crop of more than two ulcers. The patient may require difflan mouth wash and corlan lozenges or adcortyl in Orabase. Inform GP.

Gastrointestinal tract

- Anorexia, dyspepsia and nausea can occur with any drug.
- *Sulphasalazine:* if nausea and/or vomiting occurs, reduce back to the dose that was not causing this problem and increase as per protocol on fortnightly not weekly basis.
- *Penicillamine:* taste alteration can occur for up to 12–16 weeks. Support and reassure the patient. May require advice on nutritional supplementation .
- *Methotrexate:* if nausea/vomiting occurs split the dosage over the day – or two days. If nausea/vomiting persists, patient will require domperidone (10 mg three times daily).
- *Diarrhoea:–* often due to oral gold – may need to introduce bulking agents, e.g. Fybogel, and encourage increased fibre and fluid intake.
- Remember gastrointestinal intolerance could be to NSAIDs – advise over-the-counter antacids and, if it persists, to see doctor.

Headaches

- Common with sulphasalazine.
- If severe, stop drug. Reintroduce after 1 month at 2 weekly intervals.

Active joint involvement

- Joint stiffness – may follow administration of gold.

Chest symptoms

- Breathlessness with or without a cough in a patient on gold or methotrexate may be pneumonitis. Inform the doctor.

Alopecia

- Can occur while taking cytotoxic drugs, i.e. cyclophosphamide or methotrexate. If troublesome or severe, inform the doctor.

Muscle

If the patient notices weakness, double vision, swelling or speech difficulties this raises the possibility of *drug induced myositis* (inflammation of muscle) or *myasthenia gravis* (disorder of the neuromuscular junction) – inform the doctor.

Non-drug related problems

- *Septic joint:* if patient has a pyrexia and a hot red joint think of sepsis and inform doctor.
- *Neck instability:* sudden onset of weakness in hands and legs. Recent onset of bladder and/or bowel incontinence – inform doctor.
- *Early shingles:* if patient is on immunosuppressants they may need antiviral therapy. Stop cytotoxic medication temporarily until shingles has cleared.

Patients who require blood pressure recording

- Patients receiving cyclosporin: record blood pressure weekly for 4 weeks and then monthly. If systolic over 160 or diastolic over 100, inform doctor.
- Patients who present (first time) with protein +++ or haematuria +++: record blood pressure. if blood pressure >160/100, inform doctor.

References

Adamson RH, Seiber SM (1981) Chemically induced leukaemia in humans. Environmental Health Perspective 39: 93–103.

Alarcon ES, Tracy IC, Blackburn WD (1989) Methotrexate in rheumatoid arthritis: toxic effects is the major factor in limiting long term tréatment. Arthritis and Rheumatism 32: 671–6.

Arluke A (1980) Judging drugs: patients' conceptions of therapeutic efficacy in the treatment of arthritis. Human Organisation 39: 84–7.

Bacon P (1987) Vasculitis – clinical aspects and therapy. Medical Scandinavian Supplement 715: 157–63.

Baker GL, Leahl LE, Zee BC et al. (1987) Malignancy following treatment of rheumatoid arthritis with Cyclophosphamide long term case control follow up study. American Journal of Medicine 83: 1–9.

Bax D, Amos R (1986) Sulphasalazine in rheumatoid arthritis; desensitising the patient with a skin rash. Annals of the Rheumatic Diseases 450: 139–40.

Benjamin SJ, Ishale KG, Zimmerman HJ et al. (1981) Phenylbutazone liver injury: a clinical pathologic survey of 23 cases and review of the literature. Hepatology 1: 255–63.

Benner P (1984) From novice to expert. Excellence and power in clinical nursing practice. Menlo Park, CA: Addison-Wesley.

Berg KJ, F^rre O, Dj^seland O et al. (1989) Renal side effects of high and low cyclosporin A doses in patients with rheumatoid arthritis. Clinical Nephrology 31: 232–8.

Birnie G, Mcleod T, Watkinson G (1981) Incidence of sulphasalazine induced male infertility. Gut 22: 452–5.

Bradley LA (1989) Adherence with treatment regimes among adult rheumatoid arthritis patients: current status and future directions. Arthritis Care and Research 2: 33–9.

Cannon GW, Ward JR, Clegg DO et al. (1983) Acute lung disease associated with low dose pulse methotrexate therapy in patients with rheumatoid arthritis. Arthritis and Rheumatism 26(10): 1269–74.

Cannon W, McCall S, Cole BC et al. (1990) Effects of indomethacin, cyclosporin, cyclophosphamide and placebo on collagen induced arthritis of mice. Agents and Actions 29: 315–23.

Champion G, Graham G, Zeigler J (1990) The gold complexes In: Brookes P (Ed) Slow acting anti-rheumatic drugs and immunosuppressives. Baillière's Clinical Rheumatology. London: Baillière Tindall.

Clarke P, Tugwell P, Bennett K and Bombardier C (1989) Meta-analysis of injectible gold in rheumatoid arthritis. Journal of Rheumatology 16: 442.

Clegg DO, First DE, Toleman KG, Bogue E (1989) Acute reversible hepatic failure associated with methotrexate treatment of rheumatoid arthritis. Journal of Rheumatology 16: 1123–6.

Cook R (1996) Urinalysis:ensuring accurate urine testing. Nursing Standard 10(46): 49–53.

Crisp AJ, Armstrong RD, Grahame R et al. (1982) Rheumatoid lung disease, pneumothorax and eosinophilia. Annals of Rheumatic Disease 41: 137.

Daltroy LH (1993) Doctor–patient communication in rheumatological disorders. In: Newman S, Shipley M (Eds). Psychological Aspects of Rheumatic Disease. Baillière's Clinical Rheumatology. London: Baillière Tindall.

Day R (1994) Pharmacologic approaches: SAARDI. In Klippel J, Dieppe P (eds) Rheumatology. London: Mosby Year-Book Europe.

Donovan J (1991) Patient education and the consultation – the importance of lay beliefs Annals of Rheumatic Diseases 50: 418–21.

Dougados M, Awada H, Amor B (1988) Cyclosporin in rheumatoid arthritis: A double blind placebo controlled study in 32 patients. Annals of the Rheumatic Diseases 47: 127–33.

Elderman J, Davis P, Owen ET (1983) Prevalence of eosinophilia during gold therapy for rheumatoid arthritis. Journal of Rheumatology 10: 121–3.

Farr M, Scott D, Bacon P (1986) Side effect profile of 200 patients with inflammatory arthritis treated with sulphasalazine. Drugs 32 (suppl): 49–53.

Fernandes L, Sullivan S, McFarlene JG et al. (1979) Studies on the frequency and pathogenesis of liver involvement in RA. Annals of Rheumatic Diseases 38: 501.

Furst DE (1988) The basis for variability of response to anti-rheumatic drugs. In Brooks P (ed.) Anti Rheumatic Drugs. Baillière's Clinical Rheumatology. London: Baillière Tindall.

Furst DE, Clements PJ (1994) Pharmacologic approaches. SAARDII. In: Klippel J, Dieppe P (eds) Rheumatology. London: Mosby Year-Book Europe.

Ganley CJ, Paget SA, Reidenberg MM (1989) Increased renal tubular cell excretion by patients receiving chronic therapy with gold and with non steroidal anti-inflammatory drugs. Clinical Pharmacology and Therapeutics 46: 51–5.

Golding D (1981) Problems in Arthritis and Rheumatism. Philadelphia: FA Davis.

Henderson A (1994) Power and knowledge in nursing practice. Journal of Advanced Nursing 20: 935–9.

Higgins C (1996) Leucocytes and the value of the differential count test. Nursing Times 92(20): 34–5.

Hill J (1994) An evaluation of the effectiveness safety and acceptability of a nurse practitioner in a rheumatology outpatient clinic. British Journal of Rheumatology 33: 283–8.

Joyce D (1990) D-Pencillamine In: Brooks P (Ed) Slow Acting Ant Rheumatic Drugs and Immunosuppressives. Baillière's Clinical Rheumatology. London: Baillière Tindall.

Kahn MF, Arlet J, Block-Mitchel J et al. (1979) Acute leukaemias after treatment with cytotoxic drugs in rheumatology. Nouvelle Press Medical 8: 1393–7.

Kaplan RL, Waite DH (1978) Progressive interstitial lung disease from prolonged methotrexate therapy. Archives of Dermatology 114: 1800–2.

Kay A (1979) Myelotoxicity of D–penicillamine. Annals of the Rheumatic Diseases 38: 232–6.

Kay A (1986) European league against rheumatism study of adverse reactions to D–penicillamine. British Journal of Rheumatology 25: 193–8.

Kay A (1989) Monitoring of slow acting remission inducing drugs. British Journal of Rheumatology 28: 239–41.

Kay A, Puller T (1992) Variations among rheumatologists in prescribing and monitoring of disease modifying anti-rheumatoid drugs. British Journal of Rheumatology 31: 477–83.

Kinlen LJ, Sheil AGR, Peto J, Doll R (1979) Collaborative United Kingdom–Australian study of cancer in patients treated with immunosuppressive drugs. British Medical Journal 2: 1461–6.

Klein R (1974) Notes towards a theory of patient involvement. Ottawa: Canadian Public Health Association.

Kowal A, Carstens Jr JH, Schinitzer TJ (1990) Cyclosporin in rheumatoid arthritis. In Furst DE, Wenblatt ME (eds) Immuomodulators in the rheumatic diseases. New York: Marcel Dekker.

Kremer JM, Joong KL (1986) The safety and efficacy of the use of methotrexate in long term therapy for rheumatoid arthritis. Arthritis and Rheumatism 29: 822–31.

Le Gallez P (1988) Teratogenesis and drugs for rheumatic disease. Nursing Times 81 (27): 41–4.

Leonard PA, Bienz SR, Clegg DD and Ward JR (1987) Haematuria in patients with rheumatoid arthritis receiving gold and penicillamine. Journal of Rheumatology 14: 55–9.

Levine ME (1973) Introduction to Clinical Nursing. Philadelphia: FA Davis.

Leyland MJ, Cunningham JL, Delamore IW, Price DA (1974) A pharmacokinetic study of phenylbutazone-associated hypoplastic anaemia. British Journal of Haematology 28: 142–3.

Liang MH (1989) Compliance and quality of life: confessions of a difficult patient. Arthritis Care and Research 2: 71–4.

Lockie LM, Smith DM (1988) Forty-seven years experience with gold therapy in 1,019 rheumatoid arthritis patients. Seminars in Arthritis and Rheumatism 14: 238–46.

Lorig K, Konko L, Gonzalez V (1987) Arthritis patient education: a review of the literature. Patient Education and Counselling 10: 207–52.

Luqmani RA, Palmer RG, Bacon PA (1990) Slow acting anti-rheumatic drugs and immunosuppressives. In Brooks P (ed.) Baillière's Clinical Rheumatology. London: Baillière Tindall.

Malin N, Teasdale K (1991) Caring versus empowerment consideration for nursing practice. Journal of Advanced Nursing 16: 657–62.

Matteson EL, Cohen MD, Conn DL (1994) Rheumatoid arthritis clinical features and systemic involvement. In Klippel J, Dieppe P (Eds) Rheumatology. London: Mosby Year-Book Europe.

Newman S, Fitzpatrick R, Revenson T, Skevington S, Williams G (1996) Understanding Rheumatoid Arthritis. London: Routledge.

O'Brien WM, Bagley GF (1985) Rare adverse reactions to non-steroidal anti-inflammatory drugs. Journal of Rheumatology 12: 785–90.

Oka M, Vainio U (1966) Effects of pregnancy on the prognosis and serology of rheumatoid arthritis. Rheumatology Scandinavia 12(47): 7.

Oppenheim JJ, Koacs EJ, Matsushima M (1986) There is more than one interleukin-1. Immunology Today 7: 45–56.

Palmer RG, Denman AM (1984) Malignancies induced by chlorambucil. Cancer Treatment Reviews. 11: 121–9.

Parrish RS, Franco AE, Schur PH (1971) Rheumatoid arthritis associated with eosinophilia. Annals of Internal Medicine 75: 199.

Penny WJ, Knight RK, Rees AM et al. (1982) Obliterative bronchiolitis in RA. Annals of Rheumatic Diseases 41: 469.

Phelan MJ, Byrne J, Campbell A, Lynch MF (1992) A profile of the rheumatology nurse specialist in the United Kingdom. British Journal of Rheumatology 31: 858–9.

Pincus T, Olsen NJ, Russel JI et al. (1990) Multicentre study of recombinant human erythropoietin in correction of anaemia in rheumatoid arthritis. American Journal of Medicine 89: 161–8.

Potts MK, Mazzuca SA, Brandt KD (1986) Views of patients and physicians regarding the importance of various aspects of arthritis treatment. Correlations with health status and satisfaction. Patient Education and Counselling 8: 124–5.

Pounder R, Craven E, Henthorn J, Bannatyne J (1973) Red cell abnormalities associated with sulphasalazine maintenance therapy for ulcerative colitis. Gut 16: 181–5.

Powell J (1991) Reflections and the evaluation of experience prerequisite for therapeutic practice. In McMahon R (ed.) Nursing as Therapy. London: Chapman and Hall.

Puller T, Hunter J, Capell Ha (1987) Sulphasalazine and hepatic transaminases. Annals of the Rheumatic Disease 46: 421–4.

Richardson A (1992) Rheumatoid arthritis in pregnancy. Nursing Standard 6(45): 25–8.

Rossman M, Bertino JR (1973) Azathioprine. Annals of Internal Medicine 79: 694–700.

Ryan S (1995) Nutrition and the rheumatoid patient. British Journal of Nursing 4(3): 132–6.

Ryan S (1996) Living with rheumatoid arthritis: a phenomenological exploration. Nursing Standard 10(41): 45–8.

Ryan S (1997) Nurse led drug monitoring in the rheumatology clinic. Nursing Standard 11(24): 45–47.

Sambrook PN, Browne CD, Champion GD et al. (1982) Terminations of treatment with gold sodium thiomalate in rheumatoid arthritis. Journal of Rheumatology 9: 932–4.

Samuels B, Lee JC, Engleman EP et al. (1977) Membranous nephropathy in patients with RA: relationship to gold therapy. Medicine 57: 319.

Schilsky RL, Lewis BJ, Sherins RJ, Young RC (1980) Gonadal dysfunction in patients receiving chemotherapy for cancer. Annals of Internal Medicine 93: 109–14.

Segal R, Yaron M, Tartakowsky B (1990) Methotrexate: mechanism of action in rheumatoid arthritis. Seminars in Arthritis and Rheumatism 20: 190–9.

Shiroky JB, Yodum DE, Wilder RL, Klippel JH (1989) Experimental basis of innovative therapies of rheumatoid arthritis. In Cruse JM and Lewis RE (eds) Therapy of Autoimmune Diseases. Basel: Karger.

Smith P (1992) The emotional labour of nursing. Nursing Times 84(44): 50–1.

Stein HB, Schroder ML, Dillion AM (1986) Penicillamine induced proteinuria. Risk factors. Seminars in Arthritis and Rheumatism 15: 282–7.

Talaro K, Talaro A (1993) Foundations in Microbiology. Dubuque, IA: Brown.

Thierry FX, Verner I, Dueymas JM et al. (1989) Acute renal failure after high dose methotrexate therapy. Nephrology 51: 416–17.

Thompson PW, Morgan CJ, Audrey Fletcher S (1992) Rheumatology monitoring clinics In Scott DL (ed.) The Course and Outcome of Rheumatoid Arthritis. Baillièreis Clinical Rheumatolgy. London: Baillière Tindall.

Thorne C, Urowitz MB, Wanless I et al. (1982) Liver disease in Felty's syndrome. American Journal of Medicine 73(1): 35–40.

Tones K (1991) Health promotion – empowerment and the psychology of control. Journal of the Institute of Health Education 29(1): 17–25.

Tugwell P, Bombardier C, Gent M et al. (1990) Low dose cyclosporin versus placebo in patients with rheumatoid arthritis Lancet 335: 1051–5.

Tydd T, Dyer N (1976) Sulphasalazine lung. Medical Journal of Australia 1: 570–3.

UKCC (1992) The Scope of Professional Practice. London: United Kingdom Central Council for Nursing Midwifery and Health Visiting.

UKCC (1993) Standards for Records and Record Keeping. London: United Kingdom Central Council for Nursing, Midwifery and Health visiting.

Wilke WS, Mackenzie AH (1986) Methotrexate therapy in rheumatoid arthritis: current status. Drugs 32: 103–13.

Wilson Barnett J (1984) Key Factors in Nursing. The 4th Winifred Raphael Memorial
    Lecture. London: Royal College of Nursing.
Yan A, Davies P (1990). Gold induced marrow suppression: a review of 10 cases. Journal
    of Rheumatology 17: 47–51.
Zarday Z, Ueith FJ, Gleidman ML, Sobeman R (1972) Irreversible liver damage after
    azathioprine. Journal of the American Medical Association 222: 690–1.

Part 4
Patient education and adherence to drug therapy

JACKIE HILL

Learning objectives

After reading the chapters in Part 4 you should be able to:

- define patient education
- underpin practice with appropriate theoretical models
- describe the role of the nurse in patient education
- select suitable topics and methods of delivering patient education
- compile written information sheets
- discuss interventions that enhance adherence to medication regimes
- assess the effectiveness of a patient education programme.

4.1 Definitions of patient education

It may not be immediately obvious why a book about drug therapy should contain a substantial section on patient education. Drug therapy plays a major role in the management of many rheumatic diseases, but therapeutic benefit is only achieved if the patient actually takes the prescribed drugs. Non-adherence, also known as non-compliance, is a common problem associated with a variety of factors, one of which is lack of knowledge. Amongst its other attributes, patient education addresses this knowledge deficit and enables patients to make informed decisions about their own management. A partnership approach to decision-making between the practitioner and the patient not only empowers patients, it also encourages them to adhere to their medication regime as they are in part responsible for the choice of treatment.

The term 'patient education' has been used for many years, but the process is not static and has evolved over time. These changes have inevitably led to alterations in the definition of patient education. Pre-1970s definitions concentrated on the transfer of information about the body and its workings from physician to the patient. However, it became apparent that the biomedical model of care, in which a person's health is considered to be the responsibility of health professionals and the public health system, requiring little contribution from the individual patient, have little to offer those with chronic disease (Callahan and Pincus 1997). This led to a change of emphasis during the 1970s, and the focus changed from information transfer to 'self-care' (Levin 1986). As the process progressed, definitions incorporated extended information transfer and promoted self-responsibility (Bauman et al. 1998).

In the US the task force of the National Arthritis Advisory Board has developed a set of standards for arthritis patient education, which defines it as:

organized learning experiences designed to facilitate voluntary adoption of
behaviours or belief conducive to health. It is a set of planned educational activities that are separate from clinical patient care. The activities of a patient
education program must be designed to attain goals the patient has participated
in formulating. The primary focus of these activities includes acquisition of
information, skills, beliefs and attitudes which impact on health status, quality
of life, and possibly health care utilization (Burckhardt 1994).

Lorig (1996) has pointed out that modern definitions of patient
education make no mention of improving knowledge. Activities
aimed at improving knowledge are patient teaching and she thereby
makes a distinction between this and patient education. However, in
practice, teaching patients and increasing their knowledge of their
disease and treatments is an integral part of an effective patient
education programme.

Patient education has evolved into a complex process and it is
suggested that the simplest working definition is a modified version
of that stated by Lorig (1996):

> any set of planned educational activities designed to improve the patient's
> health behaviours and through this their health status and ultimately their long
> term outcome. (Hill 1997)

Useful theories and models

The mention of theories can deter many nurses, but theory can aid
our practice by providing a very helpful insight as to why particular
procedures work. A theory can be defined as a set of hypotheses
related by logical argument to explain connected phenomena in
general terms. Theories do not tell us what to do or how to do things,
but they can help to guide best practice. Models are based on theories and act as a skeletal framework on which to build. They have
practical use as they provide a formal structure that serves as an *aide-
mèmoire* thus helping to ensure consistency of practice.

The most successful patient education programmes are those that
are underpinned by a combination of theories and models (Lorig
1996). The most difficult part is choosing the one that is most appropriate for the client group!

A number of theories are relevant to patient education, in particular those that originate in the fields of:

- adult education
- communication
- sociology
- psychology.

Each has something to offer and perhaps the most successful programmes are those that incorporate something from each.

One of the underlying aims of patient education is to bring about health-enhancing behaviours, and so theories and models that are grounded in behaviour change are particularly appropriate. Many experts working in the field of patient education advocate a working knowledge of the following:

- learned helplessness theory
- stress and coping theory
- health belief model
- self-efficacy theory.

Learned helplessness theory

Seligman developed the learned helplessness theory in 1975. His research with animals showed that those receiving repeated electric shocks, however they reacted to them, subsequently became helpless and unresponsive. This work was later adapted to human behaviour, and implies that believing that one has no control over one's life leads to feelings of increased helplessness and depression. An example would be a patient who has rheumatoid arthritis for whom many of the DMARDs have produced severe side effects or have been non-efficacious. They begin to expect all subsequent drug therapy to fail and so do not feel it worth adhering to their treatment regimes. Repeated failure leads them to doubt their ability to control their disease and so they come to believe that their actions can have no effect on their eventual health status. This leads to a passive state, leaving them unwilling or unable to make behavioural changes. Patients who enter this state of 'learned helplessness' show the characteristics of:

- lack of cognition
- poor motivation
- inaction.

Stress and coping theory

One of the key elements of nursing is to help patients to cope with their illness (Wilson Barnett 1984). This is particularly relevant when nursing patients with rheumatic diseases, as they are chronic, incurable, potentially disabling and life altering. It almost inevitable that these patients experience stress and coping deficits, and so stress and coping theory is relevant to rheumatological patient education.

Lazarus and Folkman (1984) have described coping as 'a set of cognitive and behavioural responses to events perceived as stressful'. Humans constantly change their cognition and behaviours to enable them to manage specific external and/or internal demands that they see as taxing or exceeding their resources. As new situations arise, their response changes, and coping strategies will only be employed if the person feels that the threat is a danger to them (Figure 4.1).

Each person perceives a given situation differently; what is a stressor or threat to one person may not worry his or her neighbour. This is evident when patients with rheumatoid arthritis are offered DMARDs and are told of the potential side effects. Some patients are keen to try them whatever the hazards, whereas others see the side effects as more problematic than their disease. The patients' appraisal of what comprises a 'stressor' and their individual response to it is an important factor to be borne in mind when delivering a patient education programme. The educational activities must be relevant to the individual patient, or they will not be acted upon.

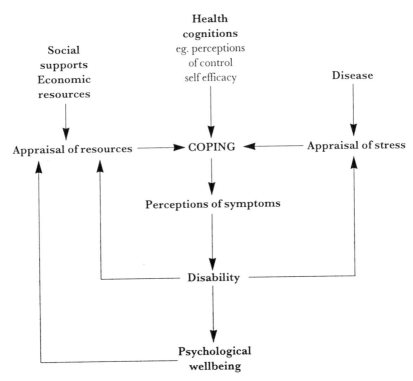

Figure 4.1 Influences on coping strategies. Reproduced with permission of BMJ Publishing Group.

Executing stress and coping theory

There is an abundance of literature on coping (Lazarus and Falkman 1984, Newbold 1996, Newman 1993). Lazarus and Falkman (1984) have identified eight discrete methods:

- confronting
- distancing
- self-control
- seeking social support
- accepting responsibility
- escape-avoidance
- problem solving
- positive reappraisal.

These and others are discussed in more detail by Lorig (1996), pp. 208–11.

Newbold (1996) suggests that patients tend to cope in two distinct ways, using problem focused or emotion focused coping strategies.

- *Problem focused strategies* are based on the acquisition of knowledge about the stressor. This encourages the belief that the stressor can be controlled and its effect modified, avoided or minimised.
- *Emotion focused coping* is based on the elimination of any undesirable feelings which follow on from the experience of the stressor (Auerbach 1989).

Coping strategies should be an inherent part of patient education programmes, but they need to be tailored to the individual concerned. Their effectiveness should be assessed, and if they are not shown to meet the patient's needs, new strategies should be explored.

Health belief model

The health belief model is one of the oldest and most widely used educational models, originally hypothesised by Becker (1974). It postulates that an individual's behaviour is based on a combination of the perception of threat and the expectation of benefit.

Patients will only change their behaviour if they believe that:

- they are susceptible to threat and that the threat has severe consequences, or

- a new behaviour will be beneficial, they are capable of carrying out the behaviour change and the cost does not outweigh the benefits.

The respect, intimacy and reciprocity within the nurse/patient relationship enables the nurse to perceive the patients as unique individuals each with their own knowledge, belief values and experience. These three aspects must be incorporated into any system of care, including patient education programmes.

People who have rheumatic diseases are usually adults whose own experience is one of their major resources and in general, they do not accept advice unless it is justifiable and makes sense to them. It is therefore inappropriate to apply didactic learning and teaching models developed to pass knowledge from teacher to child; a more interactive patient/practitioner model is advocated as being the most successful when working with adults.

The patients' perceptions are paramount and must be considered when choosing a model. This was highlighted in a study carried out in 1989 in which only 6 out of 32 patients adhered to the number of drugs prescribed by their GP. The other 26 compared their perceptions of the potential side effects and efficacy with their symptoms, and made their own judgement on the required dosage. The study recommended a shift of emphasis from didactic programmes to more informal methods of patient education (Donovan et al. 1989).

Self-efficacy theory

Self-efficacy refers to a person's confidence in their ability to perform a specific task or achieve a particular objective (Bandura 1977). Self-efficacy is a dimension of the cognitive part of social learning theory, which postulates that the interplay between physiological, social/physical environment and the individuals' cognition of their disease results in health-enhancing behaviours (Bandura 1986).

People who exhibit a high degree of self-efficacy believe that what they do can make a positive difference. This is especially important in the context of patient education, as increases in self-efficacy are thought to bring about increases in appropriate health behaviours and health outcomes (Lorig and Holman 1993, Taal et al. 1993, Davis et al. 1994).

Patients who demonstrate a high degree of self-efficacy, when confronted with a stressor, are more likely to maintain a positive sense of wellbeing and so undertake constructive coping strategies.

They are also more likely to be motivated and expend large amounts of effort on their task and persist with it. However, self-efficacy is behaviour specific. For instance patients may believe that they can control their pain, but have little expectation of controlling their sleep pattern. This is highlighted by Strecher et al. (1986) who points out that self-efficacy is not an independent personality characteristic; the individuals' expectation of efficacy will vary according to the task that confronts them. It is therefore inappropriate to characterise individuals as high or low exhibitors of self-efficacy. There is no such thing as an *efficacious person*!

It is important to understand the difference between peoples' outcome expectation and their self-efficacy expectation. Taal et al. (1996) describes them as follows:

- *Outcome expectation* is a person's estimate that a recommended behaviour will have a beneficial effect.
- *Self-efficacy expectation* is a belief in one's ability to successfully execute the behaviour required to produce a desired outcome.

For instance, patients with rheumatoid arthritis may believe that exercise will improve the outcome of their disease, but they may also have serious doubts about their ability to carry out the exercise. In this scenario, it is unlikely that the patients' behaviour will change even though they believe that the exercise would help them.

It is crucial to emphasise that it is the individuals' *perception* of their self-efficacy skills rather than their actual capabilities that are important. Bandura (1986) has stated that 'perceived self-efficacy is a significant determinant of human functioning that operates partially independently of underlying skills'.

Changing self-efficacy

Changes in self-efficacy can bring about changes in:

- behaviour
- cognitive related states such as anxiety, depression and pain.

This makes it very relevant to patient education programmes designed for those with a rheumatic disease.

It is possible to improve peoples' expectation of their self-efficacy, and four efficacy enhancing mechanisms have been described by Bandura (1986). They are:

- mastery of skills
- modelling
- social persuasion
- reinterpretation of physiological state.

Mastery of skills

Mastery – successfully achieving proficiency in a skill – is a powerful tool with which to enhance self-efficacy. Failure undermines self-efficacy and so it is essential that the patients perceive skills as attainable. The attainment of new skills is best approached in a 'one step at a time' fashion. Breaking a large task into smaller more manageable tasks, starting with those that the patient is confident of completing, helps to increase the patients' expectations of self-efficacy. For instance, obese patients may want to lose weight but be anxious that they cannot stick to a weight-reducing diet. If they are confident that they can reduce the amount of sugar they take in their tea by half, this would be a reasonable starting point. Once they have successfully accomplished this task, then they can proceed, perhaps by reducing the amount of fat in their diet.

Making written contracts with themselves often encourages patients to make changes in their behaviour patterns (Lorig and Gonzalez 1992). Although the health professional can gently guide the patient, the most successful contracting is essentially patient driven.

Performance feedback is an important factor in attaining mastery (Bandura and Cervone 1983). Positive feedback and suggested changes if poor progress is made can greatly improve skills. Patients are more likely to complete their contract when they are given this kind of encouragement. Feedback needs to be undertaken in a systematic manner and it is suggested that each session could begin with an update of progress.

Contracting and feedback are considered of such importance that Goeppinger and Lorig (1996) suggest that up to 30% of the time allotted to an educational programme should be spent on these subjects.

Modelling

Patients often compare themselves with others who have the same disease. They make statements such as, 'I feel a fraud when I come to the clinic and see all those other patients whose disease is much worse than mine.' This trait can be used to positive advantage within the realms of patient education. Other patients, who have experienced similar problems and overcome them successfully by behavioural changes, can be used as role models. Modelling is particularly useful for group education and can be adapted for use in a number of different ways. For instance, the Arthritis Self Help Programme (Lorig et al. 1985) uses specially trained lay instructors who have some form of arthritis to lead groups, as it is believed that they exhibit a powerful and positive influence. Patients can also be asked to talk to classes and share their experience of their arthritis. Groups led by a health professional can ensure that the members of the class act as a support group and help each other. For example, discussing patient problems within the group allows individuals to contribute from their personal experience, thereby reinforcing the patients' position as 'experts' and helping them towards a feeling of mastery. If the stated problem is new and has not been experienced by other group members, the health professional should offer guidance.

There are, however, a number of caveats with modelling:

- Do not choose a model who is dissimilar to the group. Goeppinger and Lorig (1996) suggest that the age, sex, ethnic origin and socioeconomic status of the group and the model should be closely matched.
- Do not choose models who exhibit spectacular achievements; this will only make others feel inadequate. It is better to choose someone with whom the group feels they can relate and emulate.

Persuasion

Persuasion can have a strong influence on self-efficacy. It emanates from many different sources, including arousal of fear, social influences and communication. Health professionals commonly use communication as a source of persuasion; gentle verbal persuasion often convinces patients that they are capable of improving their performance. Having reached their goals, patients may be urged to raise their sights and make further advances, but it is important not to become overenthusiastic. Goal setting should be realistic, as patients are more likely to be persuaded that they can reach their target if it is set just slightly higher than their present performance.

Reinterpretation of physiological state

People who have a rheumatic disease endure a number of physiological symptoms such as pain, stiffness and fatigue. Patients frequently interpret these symptoms as signs that they are managing their disease poorly and are therefore using ineffective coping mechanisms. This belief is compounded because some efficacious behaviour, such as undertaking an exercise regime, can cause the same symptoms; following exercise, the patient feels more pain, stiffness and fatigue. Patients need to 'know their body' so that they can differentiate between the symptoms of their disease and their reaction to their treatments. The nurse can play a major role in this area by identifying the patient's beliefs and then helping them to reinterpret where necessary.

Purpose of patient education

The principal purpose of patient education is to improve the patient's health status and so ultimately their outcome. However, for some patients this aim is unobtainable, and in these cases preservation of the status quo or slowing of deterioration should be seen as a reasonable alternative.

Improvement in the health status of those with a chronic rheumatic disease is heterogeneous and complicated, making it unlikely that any single treatment will bring about maximal improvement in health status or outcome. For instance, successful DMARD therapy may improve the patient's symptoms and their physical well-being but will not replace any loss or reduction of range of motion or muscle bulk. The best outcome is achieved when treatments are combined, and the patients self-manage their disease and patient education equips them to make the necessary changes to their behaviours and to adjust their attitudes. This can be difficult, as disease activity can vary dramatically from day to day and so it is important that patients can tailor their therapies accordingly (Hill 1995). To be effective, patient education needs to address a variety of different situations. As well as being able to vary their drug usage according to their symptoms, patients must learn to:

• employ positive coping strategies
• regulate their daily exercise programmes
• plan their rest and activity periods.

Limitations of patient education

Patient education is not a universal panacea. Although the majority of studies have shown that patient education can change behaviour and increase health status, the literature is not entirely consistent (Lorig et al. 1987). Even when behaviour changes occur they do not automatically lead to changes in health status, any more than increased knowledge automatically leads to changes in behaviours.

Patient education is an enhancer that magnifies the effects of other therapies. The ultimate success or failure in terms of health status and outcome is dependent upon the inherent effectiveness of the treatment employed (Hill 1997). A patient may take a particular drug unfailingly, but if the drug is therapeutically ineffective, there will be no change in health status.

Effective self-management relies upon the patients' willingness to cooperate and their ability to comply with self-care activities, so patient education is a combined effort between the multidisciplinary team, the patients and their partner/carer (Figure 4.2). However, not all patients are willing to self-manage even when they have under-taken a patient education programme.

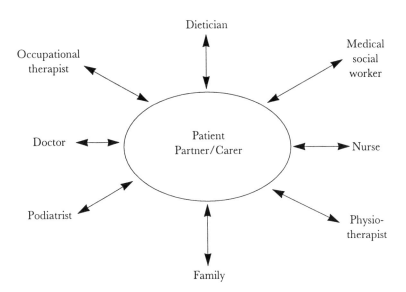

Figure 4.2 The combined multidisciplinary team.

4.2 Role of the nurse in patient education

Patient education is one of the key elements of rheumatology nursing (Hill 1995) and its importance is widely acknowledged (Hill 1998). Although patient education is not an explicit part of the majority of conceptual or theoretical frameworks used by nurses, Vaughan (1991) suggests that it is implicitly intertwined with many nursing models. The ability to self-care as advocated by Orem (1980) could not be achieved without the sharing of information and belief in self-efficacy. Similarly, Roper et al.'s (1985) ideas of maintaining independence cannot be achieved without the provision of patient education, and it is fundamental to Roy's model of adapting to stresses (1976). Whichever model the nurse decides to use, patient education will be at the core of it.

Patient education and some fundamental aspects of nursing

In whatever setting nurses find themselves, a number of underlying beliefs underpin the care they provide. These are:

- nursing is a therapeutic activity
- the nurse/patient relationship is reciprocal
- the nurse/patient relationship is one of 'professional closeness'.

Patient education and therapeutic nursing

Therapeutic nursing can be described as those nursing activities that result in a movement towards health. McMahon (1991) provides a list of therapeutic activities that can be used as a framework for therapeutic nursing which includes patient teaching as one of its components (Table 4.1). Nurses using this therapeutic model when carrying

224

out the wide-ranging role of administering, advising and monitoring the patient's drug therapy are likely to provide a better outcome for their patients than those who do not.

Table 4.1 Therapeutic activities in nursing (adapted from McMahon 1991)

Developing the nurse/patient relationship
    partnership
    intimacy
    reciprocity
Adapting the environment
    interpersonal
    physical
Patient education
    providing information
    promoting self-efficacy
    encouraging behavioural changes
    fostering coping mechanisms
Providing comfort
    psychological
    physical
Complementary interventions
    massage
    aromatherapy
Tested physical treatments
    leg ulcers
    pressure sores

Reciprocity

Reciprocity is the act of mutual exchange, and in the context of nursing reflects the belief that the nurse/patient relationship is beneficial to the nurse as well as the patient. Reciprocity is a key concept of nursing and an important aspect to encompass when engaged in the sphere of patient education. If we believe that patients are the experts on how well or ill they feel, their perception and acceptance of pain levels and their knowledge of whether or not a therapy is therapeutic, then we must also acknowledge that we health professionals can learn from the experience of our patients. This reciprocal learning can enhance the process of patient education if each party acts as both teacher and learner throughout their encounters. The incorporation of the patient's unique expertise into the nursing repertoire and the imparting of this knowledge to other patients will help to solve both current and future problems and develop understanding for future practice.

Professional closeness

Peplau (1969) used the phrase 'professional closeness' almost 30 years ago in an attempt to differentiate between the way in which peers learn together and the symbiotic learning that takes place in the nurse/patient relationship. Patients often describe their feelings about their relationship with their nurse by phrases such as 'you are not just my nurse, I feel as though you are a friend'. These feelings stem from the empathy that the nurse exhibits, and this empathy is an important aspect of the educational process. Professional closeness allows patients to feel safe and share their innermost emotions and fears. Many patients will ask questions of the nurse that they are reluctant to put to doctors; 'Will this drug affect my sex life?' or 'Can it cause impotence?' The skilled nurse can then help patients to learn about themselves and teach them how to deal with their problems. Professional closeness is an important aspect of care, but it can also become a burden to the less experienced nurse. The imperative is to meet the needs of the patient and the close relationship that develops should not be mistaken for interpersonal closeness where the needs of professional and patient are mutual.

4.3 Planning a patient education programme

Although the emphasis of this book is drug therapy, it is inappropriate to concentrate on this one topic when considering a suitable programme of patient education. Indeed, the findings of Lee and Tan (1979), who studied drug compliance in 108 patients with rheumatoid arthritis, suggest that knowledge of the disease itself has more influence on compliance with drug therapy than knowledge of the medication. It is therefore necessary to contemplate the whole gamut of educational topics and try to bias them towards drug therapy. In addition to the educational content, you will also have to consider:

* learning environment
* demographic factors
* type of programme
* teaching aids
* length and timing of the programme.

Learning environment

The environment in which patient education takes place must be conducive to learning. It should therefore be:

* quiet
* warm and well ventilated
* well lit
* comfortable.

The more disabled patients may use wheelchairs or walking aids, and so easy access is essential. A mixture of seating should be available, as partners or carers often accompany patients. Raised chairs and perching stools may also be necessary.

Patient education requires people to master new facts and ideas, and this is difficult when there are physical distractions such as pain or joint stiffness. Patients in pain will have shortened attention spans, so ensure that refreshment is close at hand in case they need to take any drugs while attending the session. Sessions longer than 45 minutes should include short breaks that allow patients to exercise so reducing the risk of inactivity stiffness occurring.

Demographic factors

Patients with rheumatic diseases are of all age groups, come from every social and cultural background and have all levels of educational ability. In fact, often the only factor they have in common is that they have a rheumatic disease. When giving one-to-one patient education this is not a problem, as the programme can be tailored to the individual. However, if group teaching is anticipated, this lack of homogeneity inevitably raises the question of whether to segregate them according to disease duration, age, diagnosis and educational ability.

Disease duration

Many people ask whether it is acceptable to teach newly diagnosed patients alongside those who have had their disease for many years. Those who have only recently been diagnosed are often confused about their illness and can be anxious and depressed. It can be counter-productive to sit them alongside someone who is clearly physically disfigured or whose psychological status is poor. Likewise, patients with long disease duration may have taken many different drugs during their illness career, some of which may have been ineffective or caused side effects. Many patients are quick to relate any problems to their peer group! This would present an improper picture to a newly diagnosed patient and would surely exacerbate anxiety or depression. On the other hand, as discussed earlier in the chapter, using other patients as role models can be a powerful stimulus and creates a very positive image of patient education.

The problem of mixing patients with widely differing disease duration has changed over the last few years as drug therapy, particularly for rheumatoid arthritis, has vastly improved. Management of rheumatoid arthritis has also changed dramatically, with DMARDs being introduced at a far earlier stage in the disease process, before physical joint damage has occurred. Therefore the best solution is probably to teach newly diagnosed patients in a separate group but to include within the team a patient who has had the disease for some time and is a good role model.

Age range

The pressure for group patient education sessions to be segregated according to age often comes from the younger age groups, who see their problems as being very different from those of the middle aged and elderly. They worry about their sexual image, marriage and family prospects and employment expectations, and many do not see these topics as being relevant to those older than they are. These fears are understandable and real, and as far as is practicable need to be taken into account.

Diagnosis

Teaching patient education programmes to patients with different types of arthritis is possible and works well in the form of the Arthritis Self Help Programme. There are, however, some topics that are easier to adapt than others. For instance, patients who have rheumatoid arthritis, osteoarthritis or ankylosing spondylitis can be taught the elements of pain control, such as rest and the application of heat or ice, in the same group. When discussing the types of drug therapy that effect pain, some, such as analgesics, NSAIDs and intra-articular injections, would also be suitable for all. However, DMARDs are not appropriate for those with osteoarthritis, and are of limited use in ankylosing spondylitis. Specific exercises are another area that can cause confusion. The vigorous exercises recommended for someone with ankylosing spondylitis are very different from those advocated for a person with rheumatoid arthritis and so teaching about this topic would be better segregated by diagnosis.

Mixed educational ability

Successful patient education requires patients to learn a lot both about arthritis and about themselves, and some patients find this easier than others. There is substantial evidence of an association between higher levels of education and knowledge of arthritis (Hill et al. 1991, Kaplan and Kozin 1981, Moll 1986). Other research has shown that a lower level of formal education is one of the predictors of mortality over a 5-year period (Fries et al. 1980, Pincus et al.

1989). It is possible to teach mixed ability classes and there are several techniques that will help:

- assess which participants will need additional help
- persuade patients to set their own outcome agendas
- check that participants understand what they have been told and ask them to reiterate
- encourage those who have difficulty understanding to attend with a partner
- teach memory aids to those who are forgetful.

Type of programme

There are a number of types of patient education programme and many have been shown to be successful. They can be delivered either informally, as is the case with opportunity education or more formally as group sessions, in fact many patients receive a mixture of both. The programmes can be taught either by health professionals or lay persons and the sessions can be given on an individual or group basis (Table 4.2). Each method has advantages and disadvantages and each patient will have his or her own preference. Whatever form the programme takes, it is important that the patients are provided with feedback about their performance, being careful to stress the most positive aspects first.

Table 4.2 Types of patient education programme

Mode of delivery	Frequency	Time and location	Taught by	Method
Individual/ one to one	Daily	Hospital ward	Single health professional	Formal
Group	Weekly	Outpatients	Team of health professionals	Informal
Arthritis Self Management Programme	Monthly	Community	Lay persons	Informal
Opportunity education	Updating sessions Evening/ weekend courses	GP surgery	Lay persons and health professionals	Informal

Individual patient education

Patient education programmes need to be accessible to the patient. One of the easiest and most convenient routes is when the patient's routine clinic consultation includes a patient education session as part of the normal management package. This is undertaken in some areas of the country, and research has shown this approach is both practical and effective (Mahmud et al. 1995).

One-to-one teaching is perhaps the most common way in which specialist nurses deliver patient education regarding drug therapy. This often occurs when patients are referred to nurse-led clinics for monitoring of efficacy and side effects following changes to disease modifying drugs. One of the most noteworthy aspects of one-to-one teaching is its flexibility. Although the programme will need to be planned, it can be tailored to the specific patient and so include topics that are important to the individual. This method of delivery also allows patient education to proceed at the pace and order of topic dictated by the patient. Before the patient education programme can begin you should:

- explore the patients' preferences about their drug therapy
- assess their knowledge of drugs
- establish shared goals
- discuss any preferred method of information transfer.

Preferences for drug therapy

Before starting any drug treatment it is necessary to explore the patients' perceptions and feelings about their drug therapy. Examine some of the practical implications:

- *Number of drugs to be taken.* Some patients are happy to take any amount of drugs; others are very wary of any pharmacological intervention. This needs to be explored. If a patient requires a NSAID and is worried about taking 'a lot of drugs', they could be prescribed a medication with a long half life such as piroxicam, which only needs to be taken daily. Drugs with a short half-life, such as ibuprofen, need to be taken 3–4 times daily to remain in the band of efficacy.
- *Size and formulation of tablets.* Some tablets are rather large and difficult to swallow and for patients who have problems associated with rheumatic disease, such as Sjögren's syndrome, or oesophageal strictures, this can be a major obstacle.

- *Memory failure.* Some patients find it difficult to remember to take their drugs regularly. This is particularly so in the case of disease modifying drugs that do not provide immediate effect. Drugs taken daily may be more appropriate for a forgetful patient than those taken less frequently.
- *Needle phobia* can pose a real problem and those who suffer from it would feel that injectable gold or methotrexate is an inappropriate option. This is also problematic when patients need careful haematological monitoring if potentially toxic drug therapy has been prescribed.
- *Side effects* are the major question in the minds of many patients. Time spent at an early stage discussing any adverse effects and how to deal with problems can be very advantageous to both the patient and the nurse. Patients value the time spent talking with the nurse and this helps to build up the nurse/patient relationship at an early stage.

All these topics need careful discussion and consideration if patients are to adhere to their treatments.

Assess the patients' knowledge of drugs

The initial interview will enable the nurse to assess what the patients know, or think they know, about drug therapy. This may sound demeaning, but it is not. There is evidence that patients have trouble distinguishing between the types of drug treatment. A study that highlighted this lack of knowledge (Hill et al. 1991) showed there were divergent beliefs about the role of NSAIDs, which are probably the most common of all therapies. Out of a total of 70 patients with rheumatoid arthritis, 15 (21%) believed wrongly that they took many weeks to start working and 11 patients thought they acted as disease-modifying drugs and stopped the disease from progressing. Approximately 30% thought NSDAIDs such as diclofenac, ibuprofen and indomethacin could induce remission. The majority of patients were taking analgesics: 36% thought these should take with food, and 33% believed that analgesics should only be taken for severe pain. The findings of this study were in keeping with other research (Kay and Punchak 1988, Mahmud et al. 1995).

Assessing knowledge can be undertaken formally, using a questionnaire such as the Patient Knowledge Questionnaire (Hill et al. 1991), or informally by discussion and questions. Obtaining the information by questionnaire has the advantage of producing numerical data that is easier to use as a comparator when assessing the effectiveness of teaching. Having made an assessment of the patient's knowledge base, this will act as a guide as to what knowledge deficits need to be addressed.

Establishing shared goals

Following the initial assessment, the next stage is to establish some shared goals. Bear in mind that a skilled nurse can manipulate a patient education session to include their own agenda alongside that of the patient. For instance, if the patient prefers to discuss pain and the nurse perceives the need to teach about drug therapy, incorporating an explanation of the effect of analgesics, NSAIDs and DMARDs will serve to meet both ends!

When establishing goals, one of the roles of the nurse is to use his or her skill to guide the patient and ensure that their goals are realistic. This is only possible if the nurse has adequate pharmacological knowledge. Reaching the goals is important to the ongoing process, and it is at this stage that patients should start to set down a written contract with themselves. The nurse can give further encouragement by following up the visit by a phone call to enquire if they are having any problems with their drugs and achieving their goals. It is also an opportunity to offer practical advice if they are not.

Preferred method of information transfer

Everyone has their preferred methods of learning. Some like written material, some would prefer visual or audio aids such as videos and cassettes and others like face-to-face communication. These methods will be discussed in detail later in the chapter, but the important point is to discuss this issue with the patient. In reality, many patients will be given verbal instruction through discussions, and written material or aids will back this up.

Having established this information, the patient education programme can commence. The format of individualised programmes is flexible, but it is still important to agree some kind of schedule with the patient. When structuring each session, make sure that you leave plenty of time to incorporate feedback of progress at the start each session and time to set new contracts at the close.

Contracting

Contracting usually consists of three basic steps. The patient decides:

- what activity they wish to accomplish in a given time
- their plan of action
- if the contract is realistic
- the activity to be accomplished.

This is the first step of the contract, and although the nurse initiates the contract, the patients should always choose the activity themselves. It is crucial that the contract is undertaken in a very positive manner, and the nurse can help by encouraging the patient to use positive expression such as 'I will take my ibuprofen with food' rather than 'I will *try* to take . . .'.

Plan of action

The plan of action is the key to success. It should state exactly:

- what the patients will do
- how often they will do it
- when they will do it.

For instance, patients on penicillamine who keep forgetting to test their urine may make a contract that states that they will test their urine once each week on Saturday morning at 9am. They will do this each week for the four intervening weeks before their next clinic appointment. They may decide to jog their memory by placing a note in a prominent position on Friday evening to remind them to save their urine specimen. Once they get into the weekly habit it becomes a routine part of their life.

Checking that the contract is realistic

This is the third and final stage of contracting. Once the patient has decided on a particular behaviour they wish to change and made their plan, they should be asked, 'How certain are you that you can achieve your aim?' This should be followed up by a further question: If I ask you how certain you are that you can do what you say by giving it a score between 1 to 10, 1 is feeling very unsure and 10 being totally certain, how would you score it?

Few patients have any difficulty with this scoring concept, but if they do it is worth trying a percentage approach (0 to 100%). You can be reasonably certain they are confident in their ability if they say between 7 and 10 or 70% to 100% sure of their abilities. If they perceive difficulties they will score less than 7 (70%), and if this is the case, it is important to explore the reasons for their uncertainty and discuss the problems that they foresee. Counselling skills can be helpful in this situation. Try to get the patients to offer their own solutions, but be prepared to proffer help if it is needed.

Once patients are sure that they have set an achievable objective, the contract should be set down in writing. Having completed the contract, and asked the patients if they would like to discuss anything else, the session should be closed with an overview of what has occurred during the consultation, and a review of the activities they have agreed to undertake before their next visit.

Having completed the session, it is important to document what has been discussed and agreed to. This will help to provide a clear picture of what has been accomplished and what still remains.

Although one-to-one patient education is labour intensive and therefore costly, a number of studies have demonstrated that individualised patient education programmes are more effective than rigid routine type programmes (Lorish et al. 1985, Tucker and Kirwan 1989, Neuberger et al. 1993). It is therefore suggested that this format be used wherever it is practicable.

Teaching in groups

Many hospitals and community groups have set up structured patient education programmes to be taught to groups of patients, rather than individuals. This method of teaching is becoming very popular, as it can reach greater numbers of patients and is less labour intensive than individualised programmes. However, like any other method it has both positive and negative aspects (Table 4.3). It may be that some skills such as different methods of joint protection, limbering up exercises and relaxation techniques can be taught to groups of patients very effectively. Those patients who have particular problems, requiring individual attention need to be given special consideration, and even in a group situation and they may require individual time. A generalised overview of the different types of drug therapies can be useful, but those who are embarking on a specific therapy are better catered for in a one-to-one teaching session.

Table 4.3 Differing aspects of group teaching

Positive aspects	Negative aspects
Cheap	Wide range of knowledge
Effective way of teaching skills, e.g. OT/PT	Different rates of learning
Patients meet others with same disease	Discrepancies in levels of skill
Share experiences and resolutions	Some patients are poor articulators
Social interchange	Difficult to express feelings in a group
Powerful role models	Fear of failure or criticism

It should be remembered that different people join groups for different reasons. Group participation can be a very positive experience from which many people benefit both medically and socially, and there is some evidence that patients learn substantial amounts from each other. Indeed, one study found that patients attributed the greatest benefit of attending a group programme was learning from and teaching each other (Campbell et al. 1995).

Unfortunately, there will always be those whose expectations are not met, and the best way to counteract this is to be very specific at the outset about who the programme is aimed at and what it is intended to achieve.

Opportunity education

Patient education does not have to be undertaken in a formal and predestined manner and every patient encounter should be treated as an opportunity to teach (Daltroy and Liang 1988). Short, unplanned meetings often take place for instance:

- at the patient's bedside
- in outpatient clinics
- in GP surgeries.

These short encounters can yield positive results in the hands of a skilled practitioner. A patient who is given a new drug can be asked a simple question such as, 'When are you going to take your tablets?' This will highlight any problems, such as whether they realise that it should or should not be taken with food. The ensuing conversation can then be guided in a different direction. For instance, if they are taking a NSAID at lunchtime, it is quite natural to endorse the fact that to prevent side effects, they should not be taken on an empty stomach. Interactions with other drugs can also quickly be broached.

A case in point would be if patients were taking oral iron and they had just been prescribed penicillamine. Penicillamine is a chelator and will interact with the iron causing reduced absorption of both preparations. Asking patients to state what time they will take their penicillamine and when they take their iron will quickly highlight any problems; the patient will have gained valuable knowledge and the consultation will have taken little longer than normal.

The Arthritis Self Management Programme (ASMP)

Chronic diseases are the greatest cause of disability and escalating medical expenditure in the US (Colvez and Blanchet 1981), the arthritic diseases being the greatest cause of disability in the elderly (Lorig et al. 1987). Greater longevity results in a proliferation of certain types of arthritis such as osteoarthritis, and its prevalence magnifies the social and economic consequences. Lorig and her colleagues in the US developed the ASMP in the late 1970s with the intention of reaching as many patients as possible at an affordable price. It is a community-based programme taught to people with almost any form of arthritis during the same programme of 6×2 hourly sessions over a period of months (Lorig 1996). It pioneered the use of lay teachers, many who had arthritis, in preference to health professionals to lead the programmes. As it has developed and research results have emerged, it has incorporated new ideas and ideologies (Hirano et al. 1994, Lorig and Gonzalez 1992). For instance, most programmes are now taught by one health professional and one lay teacher rather than by two lay teachers. As predicted, lay teachers have proved as effective as professionals in their teaching skills and are accepted by both patients and professionals (Lorig et al. 1986).

It is likely that the success of the ASMP owes much to its underlying theoretical basis of self-efficacy, the patients' belief that they can affect the consequences of their disease. Perceived self-efficacy, discussed earlier in the chapter, is believed to be a significant determinant of human functioning that operates partially independently of underlying skills.

The topics taught in the ASMP are similar to those of other programmes. However, its authors recognised that imparting knowledge does not necessarily bring about changes in behaviour, but that behaviour changes must occur if patient education is to be of benefit. They therefore developed their programme with an emphasis on:

- problem solving
- development of coping skills
- symptom management
- utilisation of information.

The ASMP has proved to be remarkably effective and is used extensively in the US, Australia and Europe (Lindroth et al. 1989, 1995, Taal et al. 1993, 1996, Davis et al. 1994). It is currently being used and researched in the UK by Arthritis Care.

What to teach

Whether the patient education is formally or informally structured, there are a number of core subjects that need to be addressed at some stage. They should include those that patients have cited as wanting more information about (ARC 1997) as well as those that health professionals think should be taught. A comprehensive programme should include:

- *disease process* such as aetiology, symptoms, blood tests
- *drug therapy:* how to use drugs, their effects and side effects
- *exercise:* the effects, and how, when and how often
- *joint protection techniques:* how and when to use splints and lifestyle alterations
- *fatigue:* its causes and how to conserve energy
- *pain control:* pharmacological and other techniques such as relaxation and distraction
- *coping strategies:* self-efficacy, contracting
- *diet:* its effects on health, fatigue
- *relaxation:* what it is, how it works and how to do it
- *complementary therapies* such as acupuncture, aromatherapy and massage
- *communication:* getting the best out of visits to doctors and health professionals
- *self-help:* knowledge of self-efficacy and approaching voluntary organisations
- *goal setting:* how best to set achievable targets and reach them.

The list looks rather daunting, and in the ARC survey (Bishop et al. 1997) some doctors expressed their concern that giving too much information about the diseases and drug treatment and its side effects could cause undue anxiety and stress. However, many patients are keen to know more (Ridout et al. 1986), as is their right, and so patient education programmes must endeavour to meet their aspirations.

Teaching about drug therapy

The inclusion of a session about drug therapy in a patient education programme is one topic almost universally accepted. It is a subject about which almost all patients ask questions, and it is a topic which health professionals feel they should teach!

Rheumatic diseases are both chronic and unpredictable, which means that patients will need to tailor their drug regimes to meet their day-to-day needs. They can only do this if they have adequate knowledge (Hill 1995). In addition to this unpredictability, patients who have a rheumatic disease usually require drugs from a number of different families to either alleviate their symptoms or, when feasible, to put their disease into remission. It is important that patients are able to distinguish between these different types of drug so that they can identify those drugs in which dosage:

- can be changed
- can be safely stopped
- must be continued.

Nurses usually teach patients about their medications verbally. However, the Association of the British Pharmaceutical Industry (ABPI 1987) has offered guidance about medication information for patients, and they state that written information should be given as a reinforcing instrument. This advice is echoed by patients (Donovan and Blake 1992) and health professionals alike (Arthur 1995). There is some research to show that written information increases the patient's knowledge. A study by Hill et al. (1997) showed significant increases in knowledge after patients had read a drug information leaflet. A combination of written information and verbal teaching appears to be more effective than either alone (Vignos et al. 1976).

In addition, the ABPI suggest that the written information should also be:

- brief and succinct
- in a standardised layout
- included in each medication pack.

Information leaflets should be aimed at a reading age of 9 years.

What to include

Obviously the type of drugs that patients need to know about will depend on their diagnosis. The more complicated diseases like rheumatoid arthritis often necessitate the use of an analgesic, a NSAID and a DMARD. They may also require steroids in one of their many forms, oral iron, an additional pain modulator such as amitriptyline and, if they take methotrexate, supplements such as folic acid. This is in addition to drugs that they may be taking for other common health problems such as hypertension or cardiac disease.

Clearly someone taking a plethora of drugs will have a lot to learn, and it is best to give information in small, manageable helpings because poor recall of information is an accepted problem (Ley and Spelman 1965). Anderson et al. (1979) have shown that verbal information is easily forgotten and that patients only recall about 40% of the information presented to them. It is therefore best:

• not to overwhelm patients with facts as they only remember the first four or five
• present the most important points first as they recall best what is said first
• discuss the patient's priorities, as they will remember what they believe important
• provide written back-up.

However, each drug needs to be discussed fully and the teaching sessions should include:

• the name of the drug
• its purpose
• how long it takes to work
• dosage instructions
• the timing of administration
• how it should be taken
• the duration of therapy
• possible common side effects
• what to do if side effects occur
• interactions with other drugs
• special precautions
• a contact in case the patient has a problem.

This is rather a long list, and bearing in mind the recall problems, the most common sense approach is to talk through a drug information leaflet such as the one for methotrexate shown in the Appendix.

It is essential to ensure that patients understand that they have certain responsibilities when taking drugs that have the potential to cause life-threatening adverse effects. However, the point of the exercise is to inform rather than frighten and so it is imperative to ensure that patients feel supported by the nurse and feel free to contact them if they have a problem.

When teaching about drug therapy, ask questions to check that the patients understand what they are being told. For instance, in the case of methotrexate:

- 'What day do you think that you will take it on?'
- 'What do you think the best time of day to take it will be?'
- 'When will you take your folic acid?'
- 'Which day will you be able to go to have your blood taken?'

The answers to these questions will give a indication as to whether the patient understands the implications. It is also a good idea to phone the patients after they have taken their first or second dose to see if they have remembered and to check that they have made arrangements for their safety bloods if they are being checked by the GP.

Risks and adverse effects

One question that nurses ask is how much to tell the patient about risks and side effects. A survey undertaken in 1975 by Ascione and Raven (cited in Meichenbaum and Turk 1987) showed that 75% of physicians did not wish patients to be told about the potential side effects of prescribed medication. The reason for this appeared to be the fear that patients would not adhere to their medications if they knew that they held risks. Today the climate has changed, and the publication of the *Patient's Charter* and *The Health of the Nation* gives patients the right to information, which enables them to make an informed choice.

It would be impossible and counterproductive to tell patients about all the possible side effects to each drug that they take. The most reasonable approach is to discuss the most common adverse reactions, making sure that you are reassuring and teaching them how to prevent problems occurring. In the case of unpreventable adverse problems, such as thrombocytopenia, reassurance as to the effectiveness of surveillance and the reversion to the normal state after cessation of the drugs should be emphasised.

Another effective strategy is to stress the positive effects of the drug therapy, bearing in mind not to promise the earth! Remember the nurse can be a powerful persuader whose role includes giving advice, instruction and suggestions.

Teaching aids

There are a number of techniques that will help to reinforce patient education. These include:

- written material
- videos
- audiocassettes
- computer programmes.

Written material

Although it has already been alluded to, the importance of written information cannot be overemphasised. Drug information leaflets are invaluable, and patients themselves are aware of this (Donovan and Blake 1992). There is also research evidence to show their worth in the community (Gibbs et al. 1989) and in the outpatient clinic (Hill et al. 1997). The results from these studies show that following receipt of an information leaflet, patients improved their knowledge of how to take their medications and their side effects. There is a wealth of written information already available, and organisations such as Arthritis Care and the Arthritis and Rheumatism Campaign produce some excellent literature. However, many rheumatology departments still prefer to produce their own drug information leaflets, mainly because prescribing and monitoring practice varies from area to area. Producing this material is an art in itself and thought needs to be given to:

- the purpose of the material
- the intended recipients
- the cost of the exercise
- the quality of the finished product

The purpose of the material

The purpose of a drug information leaflet is to inform and empower the patient, and enable them to share their information with their family and carers. As verbal information is easily forgotten, a hard copy acts as an *aide-memoire* that can be kept and referred to as the occasion arises. Although patients find this information useful, it should be remembered that knowing and doing are different things. One can know that an analgesic drug can help to modulate pain, but this is not always enough of an inducement to take it! Informing patients by providing a drug information leaflet will not necessarily increase their adherence to their drug regimen. However, if this activity is a component of a patient education programme it will certainly help.

The intended recipients

One of the most important factors to consider when writing information is the readership. The majority of the population is not familiar with medical terminology, and it is difficult to write patient literature without using it! However, it is possible providing the following guidelines are used (Boyd 1987):

- keep the sentence structure simple
- use words of one or two syllables
- use short paragraphs
- use lay language such as *feel sick* not *nausea*, or *poor clotting* not *thrombocytopenia*

Always be as positive as possible, using positive rather than negative language. For instance, 'do remember' is better than 'don't forget'. Personalising the information also helps: use words such as *I*, *we, us* throughout the document. The format is also important. Most authors now use a question and answer format, such as that shown in the methotrexate leaflet in the Appendix. Lastly and very importantly, include information that the patient wants to know as well as information that you feel they ought to know. Nurses should draw upon their experience with their patients to amass this information, but it may also be appropriate to undertake some interviews with patients of different ages and who have had their disease for differing lengths of time.

Reading levels

The information presented should be written at a level that is understandable to the patient. People with rheumatic disease are not a homogeneous population; they come from a wide range of social and educational backgrounds. If the information is to be accessible to the majority of patients, it must be readable by those with poorer reading skills. This was highlighted in a recent research project in which 12 out of 100 patients surveyed in a rheumatology outpatient clinic were shown to have a reading ability of children aged 7 years to 13 years (Hill et al. 1997). Although 88% of the patients interviewed did not have problems with their reading, these 12% would have had difficulty with much of the information already in the public domain. Some nurses have expressed their doubts that material pitched at those with lower reading skills will seem demeaning to those with higher abilities. Doak et al. (1996) are reassuring on this matter and state that both research and experience shows that adults find that literature which is easy to read is:

• preferable
• easier to remember
• faster to learn.

Assessing the readability of information

Once the information has been written, it is a good idea to assess its readability. The readability of a document refers to the reader's ability to decipher the text (Meade and Smith 1991). There are a number of formulae that can be applied to the text that estimate the level difficulty. The ease of reading depends upon the structure of sentences and the length of the words used within it. Reading formulae are therefore based upon the number of words in each sentence and the number of syllables in each word. Commonly used ones include:

• Flesch Reading Index (Flesch 1948)
• Dale-Chall Formula (Dale and Chall 1948)
• SMOG Grading (McLaughlin 1969)
• Fry Formula (Fry 1968)

There is little to choose between these formulae, so use the one most easily available to you. The more popular word processor packages have readability formulae installed in them, for instance Microsoft Word has the Flesch Index. This formula was used to assess the methotrexate information leaflet (see pp. 251–4) and showed it to be in the 'fairly easy' to read category. It is not necessary to test the readability of every word and sentence within a lengthy document.

Indeed, there is often considerable variation within most writings. It is usually sufficient to select two or three different sections of text. The further reading list (p. 258) gives sources of additional and more in depth information on readability assessment.

Reading formulae are useful tools but they do not negate the need for good writing, and accurate information. However, even well written, easily read material is likely to end up in the waste bin if its layout is poor. The patient needs to be encouraged to read it, and the use of an attractive, clear typeface will help. Consideration should also be given to those who have some difficulty with their eyesight, and a minimum type size of 12 point is recommended. A cluttered and busy design is off-putting. It is much better to leave plenty of white space between lines and $1\frac{1}{2}$ or double spacing looks attractive.

Avoid using CAPITAL LETTERS such as this for headings, because they are more difficult to read. If you want something to stand out try using a different style, such as *italic*, **bold** or larger type.

The cost of the exercise

Obviously cost has to be a consideration. Even a short drug information leaflet can be costly if you take into account the amount of time and effort put into preparing and producing it. If large numbers are required over a long period of time, it is important to make sure that you secure adequate funding into the future. Take into account that medications and any monitoring requirements may change and drug information needs to be reviewed frequently and updated as required.

The quality of the finished product

The information available from agencies such as Arthritis Care and the Arthritis and Rheumatism Campaign is of excellent quality in both content and appearance. It does not make sense to reinvent the wheel! It is only worth expending the time and energy needed to produce new written material if existing material is not suitable for the needs of your clients. It is always worth taking the time to review the material already published before embarking on the complicated task of producing your own.

Videos

Videotapes are an excellent adjunct to face-to-face teaching, particularly for the teaching of skills such as exercise. Videos can be used at home or shown to groups, and are excellent for those who have diffi-culty reading. They can also be used to demonstrate to patients or their relatives how to give injections. Some patients, particularly those who are in paid employment, find it difficult to attend a surgery to have gold or methotrexate injections. Being able to under-take this themselves not only saves them time, it enhances their feel-ing of independence. At present new drugs are being tested in clinic trials that require subcutaneous administration. There is no reason why patients cannot be taught to self-administer, and videotapes demonstrating injection techniques are invaluable teaching aids.

Audiocassettes

Audiocassettes are an excellent method of providing information for patients who cannot read or are blind or partially sighted. They are commonly used to teach relaxation techniques or distraction ther-apy. They are cheap, easily available and easy to use.

Computer programmes

Computer assisted learning has enormous potential, but of course not everyone has a computer. Suitable software can not only present information and demonstrate skills, it can also answer questions posed by patients. Some research undertaken in the US showed that patients who used a computer to access a patient education programme enjoyed it. They also gained more knowledge, improved their outlook on life, were more hopeful of a good prognosis and changed their behaviours when compared to a control group (Wetstone et al. 1985). This type of programme has also been advo-cated for use in the UK (Luker and Caress 1989), as it allows the patient to access information in whatever order and time that they require it. This freedom of choice empowers the patient rather than the educator and will be seen by some nurses as a positive move towards self-care, but by others as a threat to their authority.

Optimum timing of patient education

The greatest reduction in disability may be achieved by early inten-sive intervention (DeVellis and Blalock 1993), but there is a dichotomy within the realms of rheumatology about when to commence patient education. There are occasions when sharing information at the wrong time can make the situation worse rather than better for the patient. For instance, the nurse may feel that the patient needs to know about drug therapy when the treatment begins. However, this may be detrimental if the patient is in a state of grief or bereavement reaction that sometimes follows the confirmation of their diagnosis (Westbrook and Viney 1982). Indeed Donovan et al. (1989) suggests that patient education at this stage can exacerbate a state of depression in the newly diagnosed patient. It may be better to use counselling sessions until the patients have accepted their illness and then proceed to patient education (Hill 1997). To be able to do this successfully nurses need to develop the skills to enable them to be sensitive to the cues given out by the patient. However, this takes great skill as well as knowledge and understanding. This expertise takes a number of years to acquire and Benner (1984) has identified the acquisition of this kind of competence as that which transforms the nurse from a novice to an expert practitioner.

4.4 Patient education and compliance

There is an extensive literature on patient compliance. Most is in agreement that many patients do not adhere to their medication regimes as prescribed. This is thought by many to be a major problem, and has been cited as perhaps the most important cause of treatment failure (Henry 1985). In 1984 a literature review estimated that at least 50% of patient with rheumatoid arthritis were noncompliant with their therapies, irrespective of the nature of the intervention (Belcon et al. 1984). Other authors have estimated medication compliance to range between 30% and 70% (Feinberg 1988, Donovan and Blake 1992). Pullar et al. (1988) found incomplete compliance in 42% of patients prescribed high doses of penicillamine as their DMARD. Different authors have tried to shed light on the reasons for this high rate of non-compliance. Some of the reasons for intentional non-compliance are thought to be:

- complexity of treatment regimens
- dose frequency
- disease severity
- lack of belief in the medication
- lack of family support.

However, patients are not always non-compliant by intention. Some simply forget to take their drugs or are too busy or away from their usual environment. Lorish et al. (1989), surveyed 200 patients with rheumatoid arthritis and identified 16 reasons for intentional and unintentional missed doses. The majority of intentional non-compliance was attributed to side effects of the medication; changes in usual activity accounted for the majority of unintentional non-compliance.

Many health professionals believe that compliance is influenced by factors such as lack of information about the disease process and its ensuing consequences and the purpose and possible outcomes of treatment. Katz (1982) has stated 'one of the major factors contributing to unintentional non-compliance may be the patient's lack of understanding as to the nature of the treatment program'. There are a few studies that have explored the association between patient education and compliance with medication. Lee and Tan (1979) studied drug compliance in 108 patients, who were asked whether the physician had given an adequate explanation of the nature of their disease and the reasons for taking their prescribed medication. Of the compliant patients, 53% thought that they had been given an adequate explanation of their disease, compared with 31% of the non-compliant patients. This was a significant difference between the two groups ($p < 0.05$). Of those who thought they had received a sufficient explanation of their medication, the proportion that actually took their drugs compared to those who did not were similar. This research seems to indicate that knowledge of the disease has more influence on compliance than the knowledge of medication alone. However, this study relied solely on the patients' perception of adequacy of explanation and there was no attempt to measure knowledge in an objective fashion. Owen et al. (1985) studied 178 patients with rheumatoid arthritis and noted that poor comprehension of the purpose of prescribed medications was an important factor in non-compliance. They concluded that to obtain optimal benefit from medication, patients must be taught about their drugs.

Research undertaken by Hill and Bird (1998) has shown that patient education significantly enhances patient compliance with drug therapy and increases their knowledge of their drugs, their disease and their treatments. Patients who received patient education also perceived their disease as having less impact on their lives than controls, who were on the same disease modifying drug therapy but did not receive patient education.

Conclusion

Patient education plays an important and effective role in the treatment of rheumatic diseases, and nurses have a significant role to play in educating their patients. One of the aims of nursing is to assist patients to manage their own lives and live as fully and independently as possible. Delivering patient education programmes to our patients certainly goes some way to achieve this goal. However, patient education should not be seen as a separate function, but rather as an integral part of the practice of therapeutic nursing.

Patient education is an effective method of enhancing what we think of as conventional therapy for rheumatic disease. There is now an abundant literature to show that patient education programmes increase knowledge: Gerber et al. (1987), Hill et al. (1994), Hirano et al. (1994), Lorig et al. (1987), to name but a few. Patient education also changes behaviour patterns, for example increasing the practice of exercises, joint protection and relaxation, and improves health status measures such as pain, stiffness and functional ability (Lorig et al. 1987, Hawley 1995).

The question of compliance with drug therapy is very important, but it should be remembered that patients may have good reasons why they do not take their drugs, and they have every right not to do so. The essence of patient education is empowerment that gives patients choice. Nurses should accept that if they have educated their patients to the point where they feel sufficiently knowledgeable to make informed choices, be it to take their drugs or not, nurses have served them well.

Appendix: Methotrexate information sheet

What is methotrexate?

Methotrexate is one of a group of drugs known as disease-modifying drugs. It is used to treat several types of arthritis, including rheumatoid arthritis. It usually comes as a tablet but it can be given by injection.

How does it work?

It is thought to slow down disease activity. It can also make your immune system (your body's defence system) less effective and so it is always used with care.

It is not a painkiller, and so you should continue taking your usual anti-inflammatory tablets and painkillers.

How long will it take to work?

Methotrexate builds up slowly in the body so it does not work straight away. You may start to feel better after only 3 weeks, but it could take 12 weeks or even longer.

What dose will I take?

When you first start on methotrexate you will begin on a very small dose. This will be increased slowly until you reach your normal dose as follows:

- 2.5 mg a week for one week
- 5.0 mg a week for one week
- 7.5 mg a week for one week
- 10 mg a week as your normal dose.

A few people need a higher dose than 10 mg a week and it can be taken in doses up to 25 mg a week in some cases.

When should I take the tablets?

You will take methotrexate only once a week. You can take it at any time of the day, but you should always try to take it on the same day each week. Because you only take it once a week it is easy to forget. Most people find it best to get into a routine of always taking it at the same time on the same day; before breakfast on Friday for example.

Take methotrexate with a full glass of water on an **empty** stomach. If it gives you indigestion, take it with a little food such as a cream cracker.

How long can I stay on the tablets?

If you have no bad side effects you can stay on it for as long as it is helping. Some people have been taking it for many years.

Are there any side effects?

Only a few people get side effects. They usually occur when you first start taking the tablets. They are **usually mild** and get better in a few hours. They are:

* feeling sick
* indigestion
* diarrhoea
* skin rash
* headaches
* mouth ulcers.

More important side effects are:

* *large bruises* caused by changes in the clotting cells (platelets) in the blood
* *sore throat* and fever caused by changes in the white cells that fight infections
* *sudden breathlessness* or *cough.*

What should I do if I get side effects?

If you get side effects tell the doctor or nurse **straight away**.

Do I need special tests because of my tablets?

Yes. Before you begin your methotrexate you should have a chest x-ray.

When you first start on methotrexate your blood must be tested every 2 weeks for the first 8 weeks and then once a month. You will need these tests all the time that you are on the tablets. They check that your blood can clot properly and that your white cells can fight infections.

If your GP checks your blood, phone the surgery and ask if your blood tests are normal. If there are any problems you may have to stop taking the tablets for a while until your blood gets back to normal.

Can I take other medicines with my tablets?

Some medicines do not mix well with methotrexate. these include:

- trimethoprim
- sulphonamides
- probenecid
- phenylbutazone
- diuretics (water tablets)
- some anti-inflammatory tablets including aspirin.

Always remind your doctor that you are taking methotrexate if he prescribes other medicines for you. You should also tell the chemist if you buy 'over the counter' medicine.

Is there anything else that I must be careful of?

If you have never had chickenpox and come into contact with someone who has chickenpox or shingles, you must tell your doctor immediately.

If you catch chicken pox or shingles tell your doctor immediately.

You should not have a vaccination that uses a 'live vaccine' (polio or German measles are the most common). Flu vaccines are safe. To be certain, tell the doctor or nurse that you are on methotrexate before you have a vaccination.

Avoid alcohol, although the occasional moderate drink on a special occasion will do you no harm.

Is methotrexate safe in pregnancy?

Methotrexate can harm an unborn baby. Do not use it if you are pregnant. If you get pregnant while you are taking methotrexate, tell your doctor as soon as you know. If you are planning to have a baby, discuss it with your doctor or nurse. You should stop taking methotrexate 6 months before you plan to have a baby. This applies to men as well as women.

You should not breast feed while you are on methotrexate. Methotrexate can reduce sperm count in men.

Remember to keep all medicines out of the reach of children.

References

ABPI (1987) Information to Patients on Medicines. Policy Document, October. London: Association of the British Pharmaceutical Industry.

Anderson JL, Dodman S, Copelman M, Fleming A (1979) Patient information recall in a rheumatology clinic. Rheumatology and Rehabilitation 18: 18–22.

Arthur VAM (1995) Written patient information: a review of the literature. Journal of Advanced Nursing 21: 1081–6.

Auerbach SM (1989) Stress management and coping research in the health care setting: an overview and methodological commentary. Journal of Consulting and Clinical Psychology 57(3): 388–95.

Bandura A (1977) Self-efficacy: toward a unifying theory of behavioural change. Psychological Review 84: 191–215.

Bandura A (1986) Social Foundations of Thought and Action: A Social Cognitive Theory. Englewood Cliffs, NJ: Prentice-Hall.

Bandura A, Cervone D (1983) Self-evaluative and self-efficacy mechanisms governing the motivational effects of goal systems. Journal of Personality and Social Psychology 45: 1017–28.

Bauman A, Lindroth Y, Daltroy LH (1998) Health promotion and patient education for people with arthritis. In Klippel JH, Dieppe PA (eds) Rheumatology, 2nd edn. London: Mosby Year-Book Europe.

Becker M (1974) The health belief model and personal health behaviour. Health Education Monographs 2: 236.

Belcon MC. Hayes RB, Tugwell P (1984) A critical review of compliance studies in rheumatoid arthritis. British Journal of Rheumatology 27: 1227–33.

Benner P (1984) From Novice to Expert– Excellence and Power in Clinical Nursing Practice. Menlo Park, CA: Addison-Wesley.

Bishop P, Kirwan J, Windsor K (1997) The ARC Patient Literature Project – Brief Report. Chesterfield: Arthritis and Rheumatism Council for Research.

Boyd MD (1987) A guide to writing effective education materials. Nursing Management 18(7): 56–57.

Burckhardt CS (1994) Arthritis and musculoskeletal patient education standards. Arthritis Care and Research 7: 1–4.

Callahan L, Pincus T (1997) Education, self-care, and outcomes of rheumatic disease: further challenges to the 'biomedical model'. Arthritis Care and Research 10(5): 283–8.

Campbell BF, Sengupta S, Santos C, Lorig KR (1995) Balanced incomplete block design: descriptions, case study, and implications for practice. Health Education Quarterly 22: 201–10.

Colvez A, Blanchet M (1981) Disability trends in the United States population 1966–1976: analysis of reported causes. American Journal of Public Health 71: 464–71.

Dale E, Chall JS (1948) A formula for predicting readability. Educational Research Bulletin 27: 11–20.

Daltroy LH, Liang MH (1988) Patient education in the rheumatic diseases: a research agenda. Arthritis Care and Research 1: 161–169.

Davis P, Busch A, Lowe J (1994) Evaluation of a rheumatoid arthritis education program: impact on knowledge and self-efficacy. Patient Education and Counseling 24: 55–61.

Doak C, Doak L, Lorig K (1996) Selecting, preparing, and using materials. In Lorig K, Patient Education – A Practical Approach, 2nd edn. Thousand Oaks: Sage Education.

DeVellis RF, Blalock SJ (1993) Psychological and educational interventions to reduce arthritis disability. Baillière's Clinical Rheumatology 7: 397–416.

Donovan JL, Blake D (1992) Patient compliance: deviance or reasoned decision making? Social Science Medicine 34: 507–13.

Donovan JL, Blake DR, Fleming G (1989) The patient is not a blank sheet: lay beliefs and their relevance to patient education. British Journal of Rheumatology 28: 58–61.

Feinberg J (1988) The effect of patient-practitioner interaction on compliance: a review of the literature and application in rheumatoid arthritis. Patient Education and Counseling 11: 171–87.

Flesch R (1948) A new readability yardstick. Journal of Applied Psychology 32: 221–33.

Fries JF, Spitz P, Kraines RG, Holman HR (1980) Measurement of patient outcome in arthritis. Arthritis and Rheumatism 23: 137–45.

Fry E (1968) A readability formula that saves time. Journal of Reading 2: 513–16, 575–8.

Gerber L, Furst G, Shulman B et al. (1987) Patient education program to teach energy conservation behaviours to patients with rheumatoid arthritis. Archives of Physical Medicine and Rehabilitation 68: 442–5.

Gibbs S, Waters WE, George CF (1989) The benefits of prescription information leaflets (1). British Journal of Clinical Pharmacology 27: 723–39.

Goeppinger J, Lorig K (1996) What we know about what works: one rational, two models, three theories. In Lorig K, Patient Education: A Practical Approach, 2nd edn. Thousand Oaks: Sage, ch 9; 202.

Hawley D (1995) Psycho-educational interventions in the treatment of arthritis. Baillière's Clinical Rheumatology 9: 803–23.

Henry JA (1985) Compliance. British Journal of Rheumatology 24: 309–12.

Hill J (1995) Patient education in rheumatic disease. Nursing Standard 9: 25–8.

Hill J (1997) A practical guide to patient education and information giving. In Woolfe AD, Van Riel PLCM (eds) Clinical Rheumatology – Early Rheumatoid Arthritis. London: Baillière Tindall.

Hill J (1998) Patient education. In: Hill J (Ed) Rheumatology Nursing: a Creative Approach. Edinburgh: Churchill Livingstone.

Hill J, Bird H (1998) The Effect of Patient Education on Compliance with Drug Therapy for Patients with Rheumatoid Arthritis. Scientific Reports. Chesterfield: Arthritis and Rheumatism Council for Research.

Hill J, Bird HA, Hopkins R, Lawton C, Wright V (1991) The development and use of a patient knowledge questionnaire in rheumatoid arthritis. British Journal of Rheumatology 30: 45–9.

Hill J, Bird HA, Harmer R, Lawton C, Wright V (1994) An evaluation of the effectiveness, safety and acceptability of a nurse practitioner in a rheumatology outpatient clinic. British Journal of Rheumatology 33: 283–8.

Hill J, Bird H, Harmer R, Bradley M (1997) Do drug information leaflets increase knowledge and if so, does verbal backup enhance the effects? Arthritis and Rheumatism 40(9): S272 suppl.

Hirano PC, Laurent DD, Lorig K (1994) Arthritis patient education studies, 1987–1991: a review of the literature. Patient Education and Counseling 24: 9–54.

Kaplan S, Kozin F (1981) A controlled study of group counselling in rheumatoid arthritis. Journal of Rheumatology 8: 91–9.

Katz WA (1982) Compliance. Seminars in Arthritis and Rheumatism 12: 132–5.

Kay EA, Punchak SS (1988) Patient understanding of the causes and medical treatment of rheumatoid arthritis. British Journal of Rheumatology 27: 396–8.

Lazarus RS, Folkman S (1984) Stress Appraisal and Coping. New York: Springer-Verlag.

Lee P, Tan LJP (1979) Drug compliance in out-patients with rheumatoid arthritis. Australian and New Zealand Journal of Medicine 9: 274–7.

Levin L (1986) The lay resource in health and health care. Health Promotion 1(3): 285–91.

Ley P, Spelman MS (1965) Communications in an out-patient setting. British Journal of the Society of Clinical Psychology 4: 114–16.

Lindroth Y, Bauman A, Barnes C, McCredie M, Brookes PM (1989) A controlled evaluation of arthritis education. British Journal of Rheumatology 28: 7–12.

Lindroth Y, Bauman A, Brookes PM, Priestley D (1995) A 5 year follow-up of a controlled trial of an arthritis education programme. British Journal of Rheumatology 34: 647–52.

Lorig K (1996) Patient Education – A Practical Approach. Thousand Oaks: Sage.

Lorig K, Gonzalez V (1992) The integration of theory with practice: a twelve year case study. Health Education Quarterly 19: 355–368.

Lorig K, Holman H (1993) Arthritis self management: a twelve year review. Health Education Quarterly 20: 17–28.

Lorig K, Lubeck D, Kraines RG, Seleznick M, Holman HR (1985) outcomes of self-help education for patients with arthritis. Arthritis and Rheumatism 28: 680–5.

Lorig K, Feigenbaum P, Regan C, Ung C, Holman HR (1986) A comparison of lay-taught and professional-taught arthritis self-management courses. Journal of Rheumatology 13: 763–7.

Lorig K, Konkol L, Gonzalez V (1987) Arthritis patient education: a review of the literature. Patient Education and Counseling 10: 207–52.

Lorish CD, Parker J, Brown S (1985) Effective patient education: a quasi-experimental study comparing an individualized strategy with a routinized strategy. Arthritis and Rheumatism 28: 1289–97.

Lorish CD, Richards B, Brown S (1989) Missed medication doses in rheumatoid arthritis patients: intention and unintended reasons. Arthritis Care and Research 2: 3–9.

Luker K, Caress A (1989) Rethinking patient education. Journal of Advanced Nursing 14: 711–718.

McLaughlin H (1969) SMOG grading – a new readability formula. Journal of Reading 12: 639–46.

McMahon R (1991) Therapeutic nursing: theory, issues and practice. In McMahon R, Pearson A (Eds) Nursing as Therapy. London: Chapman & Hall.

Mahmud T, Comer M, Roberts K, Berry H, Scott DL (1995) Clinical implications of patients' knowledge. Clinical Rheumatology 14: 627–30.

Meade CD, Smith CF (1991) Readability formulas: caution and criteria. Patient Education and Counseling 17: 153–8.

Meichenbaum D, Turk DC (1987) Facilitating adherence to treatment. New York: Plenum Press.

Moll JMH (1986) Doctor–patient communication in rheumatology: Studies of visual and verbal perception using educational booklets and other graphic materials. Annals of the Rheumatic Diseases 45: 198–209.

Neuberger GB, Smith KV, Black SO, Hassanein R (1993) Promoting self-care in clients with arthritis. Arthritis Care and Research 6: 141–8.

Newbold D (1996) Coping with rheumatoid arthritis. How can specialist nurses influence it and promote better outcomes? Journal of Clinical Nursing 5: 373–80.

Newman S (1993) Coping with rheumatoid arthritis. Annals of the Rheumatic Diseases 52: 553–4.

Orem D (1980) Nursing – Concepts of Practice, 2nd edn. New York: McGraw-Hill.

Owen SG, Friesen WT, Roberts MS, Flux W (1985) Determinants of compliance in rheumatoid arthritic patients assessed in their own home environment. British Journal of Rheumatology 24: 313–20.

Peplau H (1969) Professional closeness. Nursing Forum 8(4): 342–60.

Pincus T, Callahan LF, Brookes RH, Fuchs HA, Olsen NJ, Kaye JJ (1989) Self-report questionnaire scores in rheumatoid arthritis compared to traditional physical, radiographic, and laboratory measures. Annals of Internal Medicine 110: 259–66.

Pullar T, Peaker S, Martin MFR, Bird HA, Feeley M (1988) the use of a pharmacological indicator to investigate compliance with a poor response to anti-rheumatic therapy. British Journal of Rheumatology 27: 381–84.

Ridout S, Waters WE, George CF (1986) Knowledge of and attitudes to medicines in the Southampton Community. British Journal of British Pharmacology 21: 701–12.

Roper N, Logan W, Tiernay A (1985) The Elements of Nursing, 2nd edn. Edinburgh: Churchill Livingstone.

Roy C (1976) Introduction to Nursing – an Adaptation Model. Englewood Cliffs, NJ: Prentice Hall.

Seligman M (1975) Helplessness: On Depression, Development and Death. San Francisco: WHFreeman.

Strecher VJ, Becker M, Devills B, Rosenstock I (1986) the role of self-efficacy in achieving health behaviour change. Health Education Quarterly 13(1) 73–91.

Taal E, Rasker JJ, Sevdel ER, Weigman O (1993) Health status, adherence with recommendations, self-efficacy and social support in patients with rheumatoid arthritis. Patient Education and Counseling 20: 63–76.

Taal E, Rasker JJ, Wiegman O (1996) Patient education and self-management in the rheumatic diseases: a self-efficacy approach. Arthritis Care and Research 9(3): 229–38.

Tucker M, Kirwan JR (1989) Does patient education in rheumatoid arthritis have therapeutic potential? Annals of the Rheumatic Diseases 50: 422–8.

Vaughan B (1991) Patient education in therapeutic nursing. In McMahon R, Pearson A
    (eds), Nursing as Therapy. London: Chapman & Hall.
Vignos PJ, Parker WT, Thompson HM (1976) Evaluation of a clinic education pro-
    gramme for patients with RA. Journal of Rheumatology 3: 155–65.
Westbrook M, Viney L (1982) Psychological reactions to the onset of chronic illness.
    Social Science and Medicine 16: 899–905.
Wetstone SL, Sheehan J, Votaw RG, Peterson MG, Rothfield N (1985) Evaluation of a
    computer based education lesson for patients with rheumatoid arthritis. Journal of
    Rheumatology 12: 907–912.
Wilson Barnett J (1984) Key Functions in Nursing: the Fourth Winifred Raphael
    Memorial Lecture. London: Royal College of Nursing.

Further reading

Doak C, Doak L, Root JH (1995) Teaching Patients with Low Literacy Skills, 2nd edn.
    Philadelphia: JBLippincott.
Spadero DC, Robinson LA, Smith LA (1980) Assessing readability of patient education
    materials. American Journal of Hospital Pharmacy 37: 215–21.

Part 5
The role of the community team in drug therapy

MARGARET ANN VOYCE

Learning objectives

After reading the chapters in Part 5 you should be able to:

- Discuss the advantages and disadvantages of community based practice
- Examine the role of the community team in the monitoring of drug therapy
- Describe the role of the rheumatology nurse practitioner undertaking GP based clinics
- Demonstrate an understanding of the role of drug therapy in the management of osteoporosis
- Describe ways of strengthening the relationship between primary and secondary care provision for patients with rheumatological conditions.

5.1 Shared care

Rheumatism and arthritis are major problems in the UK, affecting 7 million people. Although the majority of these people will never need hospital care, rheumatic conditions remain one of the most common groups of disorders seen by GPs. At some stage during life nearly everyone is affected with some kind of rheumatoid disorder. It is important to have a high quality seamless service, with good communication between the primary and secondary health care services.

The object of drug therapy in rheumatic diseases is to prescribe the safest, most effective drug which can be tolerated, at the smallest dose that will alleviate and control the symptoms. Pain and stiffness are the two most common symptoms of which patients complain. Drug therapy is also used in an attempt to control the disease process in conditions such as rheumatoid arthritis.

Every patient is different and therefore one drug may be tolerably effective for one patient but not for another. This cannot be predicted. Many drugs have the potential to alleviate, control and reduce disability caused by rheumatism and arthritis, but medications can also produce significant adverse reactions, occasionally resulting in death. It is therefore important that patients have a full understanding of their treatment and that stringent monitoring of such drugs is enforced, with particular reference to the second-line disease-modifying antirheumatic drugs (DMARDs).

Shared care is the management of the rheumatic patient between the hospital team, consisting of the rheumatologist, specialist nurse, occupational therapist and physiotherapist, and the primary health care team (see Table 5.1). Drug therapy in particular should be carefully planned between the rheumatologist and the GP.

Table 5.1 Members of the shared care team

Patient
Family
GP
Practice nurse
District nurse
Health visitor
Rheumatologist
Nurse specialist
Physiotherapist
Occupational therapist
Orthotist
Podiatrist
Social services
Pharmacist

- The *rheumatologist* covers a wide variety of medical disorders within the musculoskeletal system; the doctor's main role is to diagnose and establish a treatment plan to be followed in primary care or shared between primary and secondary care. The latter is the case with rheumatoid arthritis, as it is a progressive chronic disease.
- The *specialist nurse* acts as a resource for the patients, other professionals and the primary health care team. The nurse is required to be a counsellor, educator and advisor on many medical aspects of rheumatoid arthritis, particularly drug therapy.
- The *physiotherapist* provides a whole range of treatments and aims to maintain and improve function, alleviate pain and motivate the patient to carry out regular exercises to improve wellbeing.
- The *occupational therapist* provides help and support with problems of daily living and is often instrumental in enabling the patient to develop coping strategies including pacing of activities, joint protection and self-management interventions including relaxation.

The *primary health care team* provides health services outside the hospital, and is smaller and less specialised. The team consists primarily of the *GP*, the *practice nurse*, the *district nurse* and the *health visitor*, all of whom provide valuable information about the patient's family and home situation. They are often the first point of contact the patient makes. An analysis of the role of practice nurses revealed involvement with practical treatments, health promotion and disease management (Bryan 1995). When each team complements the other, and there is communication and respect for each others' roles, then good quality treatment should be available for all patients. Management goals are to control symptoms, preserve and improve functions.

Education

The most common arthritic condition seen in general practice which requires assistance from the practice nurse team is *osteoarthritis*. In one rural practice serving a population of approximately 7000 patients, 585 patients had this diagnosis (Dargie and Procter 1993). Osteoarthritis is a degenerative condition of the cartilage affecting most people over the age of 60.

Rheumatoid arthritis, which is a systemic disease affecting the joints, is less common, affecting 1–2% of the population, but it has a more disabling character and makes a greater demand for team work. Rheumatoid arthritis can occur at any age. It is destructive and unpredictable, posing many difficulties and requiring many adjustments.

Common conditions which often require less team work are *disorders of the soft tissue*, for example tennis elbow or bursitis. They may simply require an injection. It is important that practice nurses are aware of these diseases, their signs, symptoms and current therapy (see Chapters 1 and 2).

According to Bryan (1995), practice nurses are isolated from colleagues and need a forum for the exchange of ideas, the updating of skills and the acquisition of new knowledge. In an attempt to fill this need, education and opportunities for updating knowledge are provided by the hospital team in the form of study days, visits to the rheumatology unit and visits by the team to the general practice. The practice teams will then be able to support and advise patients, and recognise when side effects require a change of treatment or when the patient would benefit from a hospital appointment. The early identification of symptoms of the disease, the side effects of drug therapies, the interpretation of the blood results and their implications, plus the psychological effect of arthritis on the patients and their family, are important requisites in the education programme. The more information given to patients, the more informed decisions they can make about their treatment.

It has been shown that at least half of the information doctors and nurses give patients is forgotten within half an hour (Feinman 1997). Many rheumatology departments have produced their own drug information sheets which are a good adjunct to verbal communication. These should be clear, precise and without any medical jargon. Ideally they should be explained to the patient on receipt.

Confusion and compliance

It is important that the rheumatologist explains the planned treatment and its limitations to the patient. Donovan et al. (1989) clearly demonstrated that patients would not accept advice unless it made sense and appeared justifiable. Compliance depends on the patient's attitude, their beliefs, their health and their disease.

Role of the outpatient nurse

Nurses in outpatient departments can play an important role in drug compliance. The rheumatologist may raise or lower the dose of a prescribed drug, but the reason for this should be clearly explained to the patient during the consultation. A change in drug treatment, particularly second-line drug therapy, should be explained to the patient in detail by the nurse. A leaflet given at the time should reinforce the reasons for commencement, give the dosage, the administration of the drug, the length of time before the drug takes effect, the potential side effects, and information about whom the patient should contact if they are worried. It is often helpful if the nurse asks the patient to repeat the key facts, as the sharing of information will have different meanings to a doctor and to a patient. A drug monitoring protocol should also be sent to the GP.

Patients should be encouraged to bring a list of their current drug therapy to their outpatient appointments. This eliminates drug dosage being incorrectly administered, multiple drugs being taken out of sequence, drug interactions occurring and sometimes a course of treatment left unfinished. Patients' knowledge of which medication they were taking decreased with age; and 35% of the over 75 age group had no knowledge at all of their medications (Hopkins 1990).

Outpatient nurses are in a position to recognise the patient who is not receiving regular safety monitoring by the GP for second-line therapy. They are then able to investigate this. Outpatient nurses should advise the patient to contact their GP approximately 2 weeks after the rheumatology consultation, when the GP can reinforce the rheumatologist's requests. Uncertainties can be discussed again, and the prescription collected. Often this does not happen, with the result that the treatment is delayed.

Role of the ward nurse

Ward nurses can allay fear and confusion by explaining their drug therapy clearly to the patient before discharge, and communicating with the primary health team. Many hospital pharmacists prescribe a 10 day supply of drugs, and patients often wrongly believe that this completes the treatment.

Minimising confusion

- Nurses in the primary health care team can play an important part in alleviating confusion in the administration of drugs, especially in the elderly, by using medication cards stating how and when to take the prescribed dose (see Table 5.2).
- Poor literacy and language difficulty often impede the understanding of the drug regimes; once this is discovered, there is a need for sensitive discussion.
- Pill dispensers are invaluable for patients with poor memory, as they have compartments containing drugs for each day on a weekly basis.
- To obtain the maximum benefit, medicines should be taken in the correct way at the correct time.
- It is important that patients should not share their drugs with their family and friends, although this frequently occurs with non-steroidal anti-inflammatory drugs (NSAIDS).
- Patients should not alter the dosage of the drugs, nor stop the drug suddenly, without consultation with the doctor or the nurse.
- Many elderly patients require regular medication such as an analgesic to help reduce the pain and stiffness of the arthritis. They may not understand the action of each medication prescribed, or

Table 5.2 Medication card

Name of tablet	Dosage	How/when to take	Special instructions
Diclofenac (Voltarol)	150 mg daily	One (75 mg) after breakfast	Always take with food
		One (75 mg) after evening meal	Report any sickness/ indigestion
Azathioprine (Imuran)	150 mg daily	Three 50 mg tablets after breakfast	Take with food Report any sickness or mouth ulcers

their relationship and interaction with over-the-counter drugs. This can result in adverse drug interactions or potential serious toxic reactions.

- Many drugs contain the same or similar chemicals, and there is a danger that the patient can overdose.
- Some patients will have failing eyesight and be unable to read the instructions. Many pharmacists will print large labels to overcome this.
- Patients who have had poor hand grip often cannot open the normal childproof bottles. The pharmacist can provide screw tops or ring caps instead.
- Patients with reduced manual dexterity frequently find the packaging of NSAIDs, particularly in suppository form, difficult to open and also to administer. Eye drops also often present a problem. The pharmacist and the occupational therapist can help with the provision of aids to maintain independence.
- An increased number of tablets taken, and doses involved, often reduces compliance. Patients with poor memory may find drugs to be taken daily of more benefit.
- Many patients suffering from Sjögren's syndrome find swallowing tablets difficult. It may therefore be more appropriate to prescribe drugs in liquid form.

The primary health care team may find not only that patients have some of the difficulties mentioned above, but also that a frail, patient with arthritis may not even be able to visit the local pharmacist to collect the drugs.

Factors affecting compliance

Low patient compliance with therapeutic regimes is an obstacle to achieving therapeutic goals in arthritis management. Improvement of compliance is a prime goal of much patient education and counselling (Daltroy 1993). This area is discussed in greater depth in chapter 4.

- Compliance is often affected by *cost*. Many patients are taking a variety of drugs and they are often unable to meet the cost. An unpublished survey indicated that some women resented paying two prescription charges for hormone replacement therapy and therefore did not complete their treatment.

- Patients are also reluctant to take medication if the *side effects*, or the *taste, smell* or *size* of the tablets, are unacceptable.
- When receiving second-line therapy patients often experience no relief from symptoms for at least 3 months; if this *delay* is not adequately explained, they cease the treatment. (Conversely, if patients feel much better on a course of treatment, for example hormone replacement therapy, then they may discontinue it.)
- Many patients do not comply with the drug therapy as they are *afraid of the side effects or of being dependent* on a drug, particularly an analgesic.
- Confusion often arises as many drugs have three *different names:* the brand name, the pharmaceutical and the generic name.

Drug monitoring

At each visit the nurse in the clinic or in the practice should ask the patient suffering from rheumatoid arthritis about:

- the extent of joint pain
- the duration of early morning stiffness
- the level of fatigue
- the presence of actively inflamed joints
- functional difficulties experienced
- their coping ability

The visit is an opportunity to teach the patient about their drugs, discuss their disease progress and to offer support and advice.

Close monitoring of second-line drugs ensures their safe use and is a guide to their efficacy. To provide close communication between the GP and the rheumatologist, *shared care booklets* are usually issued to patients from the rheumatology department. They are used to record the blood results serially and monitor the urinalysis for the presence of blood and protein. This enables the rheumatologist to examine the trends of the haematological and biochemical markers and detect abnormalities in the urine, which will help them to decide whether to discontinue the drug or reduce the dose. Each book issued should have the contact number of the rheumatology department whom the patient or a member of the primary health care team can contact for advice and support. It is important that at each visit the patient shows the shared care booklet to a member of the medical team. Serious side effects can be avoided by explaining to the patients the necessity of having regular blood tests and reporting side effects early.

5.2 Community clinics

At the heart of community care is the principle that services should support people in their own home and locality (Wolf 1997). In certain chronic conditions, such as diabetics and asthma, shared management between the hospital and GP is well established (Jones et al. 1991, Thorne and Russell 1973).

In an ideal situation shared care should include:

* effective communication between primary and secondary care teams
* shared documentation in the form of agreed guidelines
* ongoing support, education and training
* an appreciation of both service commitments and difficulties (Barrett and Thomas 1992).

General practice

Most GPs will only have a handful of patients requiring DMARDs, so they are unlikely to be familiar with all aspects of this therapy, including possible adverse effects. Although the NHS management executive has decreed that the doctor who has clinical responsibility for the patient should undertake the prescribing, there is a clear need for shared management in interest of both clinicians and patients. The British Society of Rheumatology (BSR 1992) has recommended the referral of all patients with rheumatoid arthritis to the hospital setting, with the subsequent sharing of treatment between the hospital and GP.

Nurse-led community clinics

In Norfolk a weekly rheumatology nurse practitioner clinic was established in a general practice to provide the following range of services (Mooney 1996):

* physical assessment of joints

- monitoring of the safety and efficacy of drug treatment
- initiation and interpretation of clinical laboratory data
- referrals to the multidisciplinary team
- liaison between the patient and other health care professionals.

The patients were highly satisfied with this service provision. This finding was in accordance with work carried out by Hill (1997). Patients who were allocated to a nurse-led clinic within the outpatient setting were more satisfied with their overall care than were a similar group of patients attending the consultant clinic. Mooney (1996) concludes that the reported patient satisfaction could be attributed to the improved continuity of care the patients were receiving, coupled with the length of consultation time the patient spent with the nurse.

The nurse practitioner clinic in the doctor's surgery also had other benefits:

- provision of disease education for patients and the opportunity to discuss issues with the nurse
- less travelling for patients as the clinic was located in a more convenient setting with no parking fees
- patients experienced a continuity of care in their management
- the rheumatology nurse practitioner acted as an advocate between the practice, rheumatologist and patient, thereby enhancing and improving communication
- early referral could be made to other health care professionals
- if necessary, quicker access to a rheumatologist was available and appropriate investigations could be carried out before referral
- the number of outpatient visits to the hospital rheumatology clinics was reduced
- specialist advice could be provided in a familiar environment
- GP visits for rheumatological complaints were reduced (Mooney 1996).

Dargie and Procter (1993) established a nurse-led arthritis clinic in the health centre in which they worked. One of the primary objectives of this development was to provide an easily accessible service for the assessment, support, education and monitoring of treatment for patients with arthritis and their families. Additional advantages cited by Mooney (1996) included a focus on prevention rather than crisis management. The two nurses involved (a district nurse and a practice nurse) also felt they were able to make full use of their nursing skills, which enhanced their own job satisfaction. Potential disadvantages in the provision of this much-needed service were the lack of availability of community services in some areas, e.g. physiotherapist and occupational therapist. The extra time and commitment required to provide such a service could also be viewed as a drawback in economic terms, but the advantage to the patients was a service tailored to their individual needs.

The advantages of community clinics to the patient include convenience while still maintaining a high standard of care from a specialist practitioner. For the hospital one of the benefits is the devolution of some of the care to general practice, allowing more new patients to be seen in the hospital setting (Helliwell and O'Hara 1995).

Community drug monitoring

In GP surgeries most of the drug monitoring is carried out by the practice nurse, guided by protocols issued and agreed with the rheumatologist and GP. The Royal College of Nursing Rheumatology Forum has produced guidelines for all nurses involved in:

• the administration of intramuscular sodium aurothiomalate (see Appendix, pp. 284–7)
• the administration of intramuscular methotrexate.

The objective of these guidelines is to ensure that the patient receives the same standard of care and high quality service, independent of the setting in which they are nursed. The guidelines also provide the nurse with a framework for practice.

Helliwell and O'Hara (1995) found that the percentage of cases in which the standard monitoring protocol had been complied with within the GP practice was 26% for sodium aurothiomalate, 67% for sulphasalazine and 93% for methotrexate. (The discrepancy relating to the monitoring of sodium aurothiomalate concerned the requirement for an annual chest radiograph.)

Havelock (1998), in an audit of shared care monitoring, found that the majority of patients were being adequately monitored, less than 2% of patients were not being monitored and a significant number of patients were actually receiving more blood tests than had been stated on the agreed protocols.

Shared care documentation

Patients taking DMARDs or cytotoxic agents require regular blood and urine tests (see Chapter 3). The findings of such investigations are often recorded in a patient-held monitoring booklet provided by the rheumatology department (see p. 267). This booklet is taken by the patient to their clinic appointment (whether in a primary or secondary care environment) to provide a record of the safety and efficacy of current drug therapy. The success of drug monitoring via this method is dependent on good communication between the hospital and primary health care team. A hospital based telephone helpline is a useful facility to enhance the communication required, as it ensures that any member of the community team (including the patient) has direct access to a knowledgeable clinician familiar with the patient's care, for advice and support. In Helliwell and O'Hara's study (1995) there was unanimous agreement by the GPs that the shared monitoring cards were helpful. The GPs involved were prepared to keep the cards up to date and were willing to follow suggested protocols. Havelock (1998) also found that this method of documentation worked well within both the primary and secondary care settings.

GP's concerns relating to practice based monitoring

Anxieties over various aspects of GP based drug monitoring included:

- poor facilities for the collection and distribution of blood samples to the hospital laboratory
- a perceived lack of time for domicilary visits to those patients unable to attend the practice (although one could argue that it might be more appropriate for a community practitioner, e.g. a district nurse with expanded knowledge in the field of rheumatology, to carry out such visits)
- lack of clarity regarding the responsibility for prescribing and monitoring drug therapy.

One practice cited by Helliwell and O'Hara (1995) was unwilling to monitor second-line therapy due to a perceived lack of time to perform the necessary blood tests and a reluctance to accept the responsibility.

Rheumatologist community clinics

Essential features of community clinics include:

- location close to the patient's home
- performed by a consultant specialist
- provision of educational opportunities for GPs
- improved communication between the hospital and community staff (Helliwell 1996).

Advantages from community clinics in medical and surgical specialities have included:

- shorter waiting time for first appointment
- ease of access for patients
- fewer non-attenders
- patients seen by the specialist every time (Bailey et al. 1994).

Patients in Helliwell's study (1996) reported experiencing a greater satisfaction with their consultations than their counterparts attending a hospital based clinic. Patients attending the community clinic stated that their questions were always answered.

Potential problems with consultant based community clinics

- Many consultants working within the community have a minimal number of support staff, and the time spent travelling will reduce the number of patients seen per session (Barnyl et al. 1990).
- The opportunity for education as a result of personal contact between the consultant and GP is often infrequent because GPs have busy surgeries of their own (Helliwell 1996). In a survey by Bailey et al. (1994), GPs were in attendance at only 5% of outreach clinics
- Case mix disruptions may occur if the consultant sees all follow-up patients and no new referrals, and the consultant is not available for other clinical practices while in the community (Walker 1994). Although fewer patients were seen in the community clinic, with a higher old/new ratio than the hospital based clinic, Helliwell (1996) found no difference in the case mix data between the two health care settings.

5.3 Drug therapy and osteoporosis

As is often the case in the management of many chronic conditions, it is the primary health care team who are responsible for the early diagnosis and continuing care of patients with established osteoporosis (Brennan 1996).

Osteoporosis is a silent disease that can affect all age groups. Symptoms are not usually present until a fracture occurs, often as a result of minimal trauma. Bone is a living tissue and is being continually regenerated. Cells called *osteoclasts*, destroy bone and eat away areas of it, while others, called *osteoblasts*, are bone builders; they follow the osteoclasts, filling in and repairing the bone. When this process becomes unbalanced, and more bone is destroyed than is being replaced, then osteoporosis results with bones becoming thinner and more brittle.

Peak bone mass is generally achieved between the ages of 25 and 36. Following this peak, bone mass decreases by 0.3% a year. When women reach the menopause, however, bone loss is more rapid and may be as much as 5% per year over a 10-year period.

Classification of osteoporosis

Osteoporosis falls into two categories, primary and secondary.

- *Primary osteoporosis* is caused by ageing, the menopause and impaired adult peak bone density.
- *Secondary osteoporosis* is caused by:
  - anorexia and bulimia
  - amenorrhoea for more than 6 months
  - premature menopause (whether surgical, natural or radiation induced)

- excessive exercise (e.g. in dancers and athletes)
- lifestyle factors (e.g. smoking and excessive alcohol)
- dietary factors (e.g. lack of calcium and vitamin D) (Table 5.3 shows food groups rich in calcium)
- gut malabsorption and chronic liver disease
- immobilisation
- high dose corticosteroid therapy (over 7.5 mg daily)
- anticonvulsants
- heparin therapy
- genetic factors
- Cushing's syndrome.

Table 5.3 Foods rich in calcium

Food	Portion size	Calcium content (mg)
Yoghurt	150 g	225
milk (whole)	190 ml	234
milk (skimmed)	190 ml	235
milk (semi-skimmed)	190 ml	231
milk (soya)	190 ml	25
Cheese (Cheddar)	28 g	202
Cheese (Edam)	28 g	216
Sardines (tinned)	56 g	258
Spinach (boiled)	112 g	179
Baked beans	112 g	59
Bread (white)	1 slice	33
Bread (wholemeal)	1 slice	16

It is important that the primary health care team identify those individuals who are potentially at risk and discuss with them preventive strategies or management of the condition.

Investigations for osteoporosis risk

If osteoporosis is to be treated and prevented, potential sufferers must first be identified. Highly sensitive equipment is now available which can detect low bone density, a key determinant of bone strength. By comparing an individual's bone density at clinically important sites such as the spine and femoral neck against 'normal ranges', the individual's future fracture risk can be established.

- *Dual energy x-ray absorptiometry* (DXA) is currently the most precise and widely used method of assessing bone density. It is an accurate, reliable, non-invasive technique and the current best indicator of fracture.

* *Quantitive computed tomography* (QCT) systems have been adapted to estimate bone mineral content allowing cortical bone to be separated from trabecular bone. However, it is expensive and exposes patients to radiation.
* *Radiography:* 30% of the skeleton may be lost before osteoporosis becomes apparent on x-ray.
* Further research is required to assess *ultrasound measurement* as a means for assessing bone density and predicting future fracture risk.

Hormone replacement therapy (HRT)

The incidence of osteoporosis is far greater in women than in men. After the menopause, women experience a rapid loss of bone density as a result of oestrogen deficiency. Replacing that oestrogen in the form of HRT will prevent bone loss and maintain bone density (Lindsay et al. 1976, 1978, Christiansen and Lindsay 1990). Studies have shown a reduction in risk of hip and forearm fracture with long term use of HRT (Kiel et al. 1987, Nassen et al. 1990).

All women should be advised about using HRT at the time of the menopause. Use of HRT in the UK has been limited mainly to those women wanting relief of menopausal symptoms. In order to prevent osteoporosis, women need to take HRT for years rather than months.

Nurses have a very important role to play in ensuring that women receive the necessary information to make an informed choice about HRT.

Advantages

The advantages of HRT include reduced risk of coronary heart disease (Bush 1991), strokes in menopausal women and myocardial infarction. It also reduces the symptoms of the menopause – night sweats, irritability, hot flushes and vaginal dryness.

Disadvantages

One of the disadvantages of HRT is that after 5 years there may be a possibility of an enhanced risk of breast cancer (Colditz et al. 1995). The risk of endometrial cancer is increased if oestrogen alone is prescribed to patients with a womb, and therefore oestrogen combined either cyclically or continuously with progesterone is used. Nausea, breast tenderness, fluid retention and weight gain are sometimes experienced, but these tend to disappear. Migrainous headaches and irregular vaginal bleeding should be reported to the doctor. For older women the return of periods may be viewed as a disadvantage, but now period-free medications, such as continuous combined oestrogen with progesterone or tibolone (Livial), have been developed.

Contraindications

Contraindications to HRT include breast cancer, endometrial cancer, liver disease, or recent thrombosis. Malignant melanoma, known or suspected pregnancy, undiagnosed vaginal bleeding and endometrial hyperplasia will all require discussion with the doctor when considering HRT.

Administration

Before commencing HRT all patients should have their blood pressure recorded, a vaginal smear taken and a mammogram performed. HRT can be commenced at any age but the closer to the menopause the more effective it will be in slowing down or stopping bone loss. It is prescribed in various forms; as tablets, a medicated patch or an implant. The gels and sprays are as yet not as effective as other forms of HRT.

Combined HRT is prescribed to women who have a womb. Oestrogen is given to control the menopausal symptoms and to protect the bones, and progesterone is prescribed for at least 12 days at the end of the cycle to remove the endometrium of the uterus, resulting in a menstrual bleed. The minimum amount of oestrogen required to protect the skeleton is 0.625 mg of equine oestrogen, or 2 mg of oesdradiol. Oestrogen and progesterone can be given daily in a continuous combined HRT such as Premique, Kliofem or Climesse. Continuous oestrogen should be given to women who have had a hysterectomy.

- *Oral preparations* are usually well tolerated, but some women may prefer alternative routes of delivery. Generally, patients should commence HRT on the lowest dose possible and gradually increase until the symptoms are controlled. This may take time and some women will tolerate one preparation and some another.

- A *transdermal medicated patch* attached to the buttock or the abdomen is another way of taking HRT. This allows its contents to be absorbed through the skin directly into the blood stream. If skin irritation occurs, it may have to be changed every day to a different site.

- *Oestradiol coated implant* which can be inserted subcutaneously in the abdomen. This is only effective for 6 months.

Both patches and implants are beneficial to patients with malabsorption, diabetes, thrombosis or previous liver disease.

Regular monitoring of blood pressure, breast examination and mammography is recommended throughout this therapy. Unfortunately the compliance is poor owing to the fear of cancer, transient postmenopausal symptoms, menstruation, and the cost of the prescription charge of a combined pill. It is important in the early stages of this therapy that the nurses and the primary health care team should support, encourage and educate patients.

Drug therapy for patients with established osteoporosis

Pain management

Simple analgesics such as paracetamol and NSAIDs can be beneficial for chronic pain in osteoporosis. Opiates (e.g. morphine) and calcitonin are sometimes given for the intense pain of a vertebral fracture. If chronic pain is not acknowledged then the patient becomes less active, more helpless and isolated, and self-esteem is greatly reduced. Non-pharmacological management of pain is shown in Table 5.4.

Preventing fractures

A good balanced diet with calcium and vitamin D, plus adequate exercise and HRT for postmenopausal women, are recommended to prevent fractures. Drug therapy can also be used. Bisphosphonates are powerful anti-resorptive agents. They reduce osteoclast number and function and stimulate bone growth. They can increase the density of the bone by 5% over 4 years and can be used for both men and women.

Table 5.4 Pain management (non-pharmacological)

Pacing activities
Relaxation
Joint protection techniques
Aids and adaptation
Hydrotherapy
Exercise
Use of heat (e.g. heat pads)
Massage (aromatherapy)
Diversional therapy
Counselling
Transcutaneous electrical nerve stimulation (TENS) machine

Bisphosphonates

ETIDRONATE DISODIUM

Etidronate (Didronel PMO, cyclical etidronate) is a non-hormonal treatment for osteoporosis and is the first choice in postmenopausal women with a vertebral fracture due to osteoporosis. This is recommended for patients under 75 years of age and is prescribed in a 3 month cyclical pack, 14 consecutive days of etidronate 400 mg following by 76 days of calcium carbonate 500 mg. The 90 day pack is continually repeated. Etidronate is well tolerated but is poorly absorbed and should therefore be taken in the middle of a 2 hour fast away from other medication. Contraindications for this drug are severe renal impairment, hypocalcaemia, hypercalcinuria, pregnancy and lactation.

Studies of cyclical etidronate have shown long-term benefits in terms of an increase in bone density and a reduction in the incidence of vertebral fractures.

• Storm et al. (1990) found that cyclical etidronate therapy increased lumbar spine mass by 5.3% over 3 years and reduced the incidence of new vertebral fractures.
• Watt et al. (1990) found that spine bone density increased by 4.7% over 2 years and was most marked in patients with the lowest bone density. There is now evidence (Harris et al. 1993) to suggest that the beneficial effects of etidronate on spine and femoral bone density and vertebral fracture rate may be maintained after 4 years of use. The licence for the use of Didronel PMO is no longer restricted to 3 years.

ALENDRONIC ACID

Alendronic acid (Fosamax) is licensed for use in the UK. It is taken as a single 10 mg daily dose. It is well tolerated but cases of oesophagitis have been reported. Patients should swallow a 10 mg tablet when getting out of bed in the morning, half an hour before any food and with a 150 ml (7 oz) drink of plain water. It is important that patients should stand or sit for at least 30 minutes after taking Fosamax and not go back to bed. Antacids can affect the absorption of this drug. Contraindications are patients with significant renal impairment, pregnant and breast-feeding women, patients with abnormalities of the oesophagus or upper gastrointestinal problems. The side effects include nausea, dyspepsia and diarrhoea. Treatment is continued long term. It is useful treatment for older women with established osteoporosis who do not wish to take HRT. It would be potentially suitable treatment for men with osteoporosis but there is at present limited data to support its efficacy. Recker et al. (1995) demonstrated that treatment of women with alendronic increases bone density by 8.2% in the spine and 7.2% in the hip over 3 years. This increase in spine bone density is associated with a reduction in the evidence of new vertebral fracture.

CALCITONIN

Calcitonin is a natural thyroid hormone. It decreases osteoclast activity by blocking the stimulatory effects of the parathyroid hormone and, as a result, bones become stronger and are less likely to fracture. It is given by injection. As calcitonin is derived from salmon or pork, it is important that a test dose should be given subcutaneously or intramuscularly before therapy commences. Calcitonin treatment prevents cortical and trabecular bone loss in osteoporotic women, and also reduces the pain of spinal fractures. It is an expensive form of treatment with few side effects and is given for a limited period. Nausea, vomiting, dizziness and diarrhoea have been reported. In some countries it can be administered as an intranasal spray.

CALCIUM SUPPLEMENTS

It is not necessary to give calcium supplements if patients have an adequate diet, but often in the elderly this is not possible and calcium supplements are then recommended. It has been found useful in patients with dietary deficiencies and those with lactose intolerance, or where other treatments are unacceptable. The tablets are swallowed whole, chewed or acquired in soluble form. They can be purchased in chemists or health food shops. A total intake of 1–1.5 g a day is required. Calcium supplements decrease bone loss but not to the same extent as other anti-resorptive agents Reid et al. (1993).

Vitamin D

Vitamin D is needed for calcium to be absorbed into bone. Sunshine is the natural source of vitamin D. Vitamin supplements are prescribed to the elderly and to people who are not exposed to sunlight or who have had a low renal function or lower calcium absorption from the gut. The normal dose is 400–500 International Units (IU) per day, and vitamin D is often given in conjunction with calcium supplements. With advancing age there is a reduction in cutaneous production and subsequent metabolism of vitamin D which leads to a decrease in calcium absorption. A French study in nursing homes showed that 800 iu of vitamin D_3 and 1.2 g of elemental calcium daily reduces the risk of hip fracture by 43% (Chapuy et al. 1992). There is no evidence that vitamin D and calcium supplementation decreases spine bone loss or the incidence of vertebral fracture.

Calcitriol

Calcitriol is an active form of vitamin D which is needed for calcium to be absorbed into the bone. It appears to be well tolerated and is a viable treatment option for postmenopausal women with one or two vertebral fractures. It is given in tablet form but is not suitable for women with hypercalcaemia. Studies of the effect of treatment with vitamin D metabolites on bone loss and fracture in established osteoporosis have produced conflicting results.

Anabolic steroids

Anabolic steroids are rarely used for osteoporosis in the UK. Drugs such as stanozol (Stromba) and nandrolene (Deca-Durabolin) increase bone mass but there is no evidence of a reduction in fracture incidence. Anabolic steroids may be associated with androgenic side effects and fluid retention, and prolonged administration may lead to abnormal liver function tests and even hepatocellular tumours.

Testosterone

Testosterone is beneficial for men with established osteoporosis who have low circulating levels of the hormone. It is given intramuscularly at 2 week intervals, orally, as 4–6 month implants or as patches. The injection is a thick liquid and needs warming in the palm of the hand before giving. This injection is painful. One form of treatment is

Sustanon; this cannot be taken as long-term therapy as it may affect the prostate. Patients should be monitored as there is an increased risk of heart disease, and occasionally the patient may become aggressive.

Osteoporosis occurs in 1 in 12 men, usually over the age of 60, due to gradual loss of bone density, but it can occur in younger men due to an underlying condition such as hypogonadism (low testosterone level), excessive drinking and smoking, prolonged steroid therapy and malabsorption problems.

SODIUM FLUORIDE

Sodium fluoride 75 mg daily increases spine bone density by up to 35% over 4 years in women with vertebral osteoporosis, but this appears to be at the expense of cortical bone loss. There is no reduction in vertebral fracture increase, whereas the number of non vertebral fractures is increased with fluoride (Kleerekoper et al. 1991). Sodium fluoride is potentially toxic, causing nausea, vomiting, indigestion and bone pain in the feet.

PARATHYROID HORMONE

The effect of parathyroid hormone (PTH) on bone turnover depends on the use and frequency of administration. Continuous or high dose treatment causes bone loss, whereas intermittent low dose therapy increases trabecular bone density by as much as 50%, although this may be at the expense of cortical bone. PTH therefore remains an experimental treatment and there is no data on its effects on fracture incidence.

Prevention of osteoporosis

Lifestyle strategies

Diet

For optimum bone health a well balanced diet is recommended with adequate calcium and vitamin D (see Table 5.3). Calcium requirements change throughout life, and an adequate intake is particularly important during childhood, adolescence, pregnancy and lactation. Excessive caffeine, salt and fibre can hamper absorption and increase calcium excretion.

Smoking

Smoking reduces osteoblast production and alters oestrogen

metabolism in women. Women smokers tend to have an earlier menopause.

Alcohol

The effects of excessive alcohol consumption on bone are multifactorial, reducing calcium absorption, and damaging the liver and bone cells.

Exercise

Weight-bearing exercise can increase bone formation, improve muscle strength and coordination. Exercise must be sustained as bone loss will resume once exercise stops. Exercise can also improve coordination and reduce the likelihood of falls. Three 20-minute sessions of exercise weekly are required. Excessive exercise will have a negative effect and increase the risk of osteoporosis due to low body weight and the effects on the hypothalamic–pituitary–gonadal axis.

Avoiding falls

Nurses have an input in preventing falls by improving awareness, identifying these who might be at risk and addressing risk factors such as eyesight, footwear, safety in the home, etc.

Role of the primary health care team

The primary health care team play an important part in the prevention of osteoporosis by being aware of the clinical triggers, discussing HRT at the menopause, and talking to patients who have had a fracture following a minor incident. They can give opportunist counselling and advice to patients when discussing other conditions.

Finally, education at all ages is particularly helpful from the primary health care team in preventing osteoporosis. Ongoing monitoring, assessment, advice and support from the health care team is important to ensure that patients take the medication, particularly the bisphosphonates, at the correct time and in the correct way.

Conclusion

The primary health care team play a valuable preventive role, especially with regard to osteoporosis, emphasising the importance of a healthy life style from the cradle to the grave. They often have a good relationship with patients because they see them for a multitude of conditions.

It is the responsibility of the primary health care team, with the support of the rheumatologists and their team, to ensure the continuity of complex care which is offered to the rheumatology patient. What is regarded as routine in the rheumatology clinic may be rare to the GP. It is therefore important that the appropriate information is given to the patient on ward discharge and after clinic appointments, and to the GP with a diagnosis and details of medication and treatment.

A network of support and communication between rheumatology services, the rheumatology team, the district nurses, the practice nurses and other community based services will ensure consistent, clinically effective management of the patient and their rheumatoid disease. It is important that the practice nurse team utilises the rheumatology nurse practitioner in a co-ordinating role as a resource and advisor. Management of arthritis is a long term partnership between the patient and the primary and secondary health care team.

Appendix: Guidelines for nurses on the use and administration of sodium aurothiomalate in rheumatoid arthritis

What is sodium aurothiomalate?

Sodium aurothiomalate (intramuscular gold) belongs to the group of drugs known as slow-acting antirheumatic drugs (SAARDs) or disease-modifying antirheumatic drugs (DMARDS). These drugs suppress clinical and laboratory markers of disease activity and are thought to slow the progression of the disease but the precise mode of action is unknown. Unlike non-steroidal anti-inflammatory drugs (NSAIDs) which produce an immediate therapeutic effect, DMARDs are unlikely to produce any benefit before 12 weeks and often take as long as 24 weeks before improvement is attained.

Indications for using sodium aurothiomalate

Sodium aurothiomalate is used in cases of active rheumatoid arthritis.

Contraindications

Women who are pregnant or are breast-feeding should not be given intramuscular gold: likewise those who have gross renal or hepatic disease, history of blood dyscrasias, exfoliative dermatitis or systematic lupus erythematosus.

Administration and dosage of sodium aurothiomalate

The drug is given by deep intramuscular injection, followed by gentle massage of the area. An initial test dose of 5–10 mg is usually given and if there are no adverse reactions (skin rash or hypersensitivity), weekly injections of 20–50 mg are administered until a response occurs. Most patients will feel no benefit until they have received a total dose of 500–800 mg. Once in remission and providing they do not experience any side effects, patients are usually maintained on a dose of 50 mg administered monthly, but the physician may vary the dose according to the activity of the disease. If no major improvement has occurred after reaching a total dose of 1000 mg (excluding the test dose) the treatment is usually discontinued, although sometimes weekly injections of 100 mg for 5 weeks are given.

Adverse reactions

Side effects occur in approximately 30% of patients and can appear at any time during the course of the treatment, even after the patient has been successfully treated with sodium aurothiomalate for many years. They are mostly mild, but up to 5% experience severe reactions which are potentially fatal.

Skin

Skin reactions are perhaps the most common of the side effects to intramuscular gold and are usually mild. However, if they do develop, the injection should be withheld and their presence should always be reported to the physician as they may be the forerunners to severe gold toxicity. This side effect occurs most commonly after a total cumulative dose of 300–400 mg.

Rashes may be localised or general and range from minor reactions to major skin lesions. They can mimic almost any skin eruption. Pruritus or itching is quite common and is often first felt between the fingers.

Mucous membranes

Stomatitis and mouth ulcers can develop in some patients. Pharyngitis should raise the question of leucopenia. Patients sometimes complain of a metallic taste in the mouth which, although unpleasant, is not a permanent side effect.

Blood

Thrombocytopenia, neutropenia, agranulocytosis and fatal marrow suppression can develop but the last of these is rare. Bruising, particularly around the shins, can be the first indication of thrombocytopenia. A fever and sore throat can indicate the presence of agranulocytosis.

Eosinophilia may be an indication of developing toxicity but does not always necessitate stopping gold.

The drug manufacturer recommends that a full blood and platelet count is taken before each injection is given and this should be meticulously adhered to. These results should be recorded sequentially. A sudden fall in platelet or white cell count outside normal limits may be reason for the physician to suspend treatment. A fall on three consecutive occasions, even if within normal limits, should also be reported as the physician may wish to suspend or modify the treatment.

Blood dyscrasias are most likely to happen when between 400 mg and 1000 mg of intramuscular gold has been given, but can occur at anytime during treatment.

Kidney

Proteinuria develops in about 10% of patients but is severe in less than 2%.

A gradual increase in protein concentration is more significant than a single result, so if protein is detected, do not give the gold but ask the patient to return a few days later for a retest. If the protein persists, consult the clinician; it may be necessary to estimate the amount of protein excreted in 24 hours by a more accurate measure than use of dipsticks.

If blood and protein are present, eliminate the possibility of a urinary infection by collecting a midstream urine (MSU) specimen; if the MSU is negative, the clinician may decide to stop the gold.

Rarer side effects

Rarer side effects include peripheral neuritis, alopecia and colitis.

A small number of patients may experience flushing, nausea or vertigo after an injection.

The nurse's responsibility when giving sodium aurothiomalate

Before beginning the gold injections, you should discuss the treatment with the patient. This should include an explanation of what the treatment is for, how it is to be given, how the treatment will help and what side effects may occur. It is also important to make sure that the patient knows where the treatment and monitoring will take place, and who they should contact if they are unable to attend or if they experience any problems. It is always helpful to provide written information to the patient as a backup to this verbal explanation.

Before each injection

1. Inspect the skin for rashes and ask if any pruritus (itching) has been experienced.
2. Ask the patient if they have experienced any soreness of the throat, mouth ulcers or loss of taste.
3. Ascertain that blood has been taken for a full blood count.
4. Check that the prescribing clinician has seen and approved the results of the previous blood tests.
5. Inspect the skin for bruising.
6. Inquire if the patient has experienced any undue bleeding such as epistaxis or bleeding gums.
7. Ask the patient if they are experiencing any flu-like symptoms.
8. Record the dose given, haematology and urinalysis results, the presence of any unwanted effects and any action taken on the patients gold card.

If the monitoring reveals any adverse effects, withhold the gold and report the symptoms to the doctor.

References

Barrett CW, Thomas J (1992) Shared care – the way forward. Hospital Update plus 18: 7–10.

Bailey JJ, Black ME, Wilkin D (1994) Specialist outreach clinics in general practice. British Medical Journal 308: 1083–6.

Barnyl A, Dieppe P, Haslock I, Shipley ME (1990) What do rheumatologists do? A pilot audit study. British Journal of Rheumatology 29: 295–8.

BSR (1992) Guidelines and audit measures for the specialist supervisor of patients with rheumatoid arthritis. Joint working group with the royal college of physicians. London: British Society of Rheumatology.

Brennan J (1996) In practice managing osteoporosis care of the elderly. Geriatric Medicine 26(6): 1–2.

Bryan C (1995) Practice nursing – the study of the role. Nursing Standard 9(17): 25–9.

Bush TL (1991) The extraskeletal effects of oestrogen and prevention of arthrosclerosis. Osteoporosis International 2: 5–11.

Chapuy MC, Arlot ME, Duboeuf F, Brun J, Crouzet B, Arnaud S (1992) Vitamin D_3

and calcium to prevent hip fractures in elderly women. New English Journal of Medicine 327: 1637–42.

Christiansen C, Lindsay R (1990) Estrogens, bone loss and preservation. Osteoporosis International 1: 7–13.

Colditz GA, Hankinson SE, Hunter DJ (1995) The use of estrogens and progestins and the risk of breast cancer in post menopausal women. New English Journal of Medicine 332: 1589–93.

Daltroy L (1993) Doctor patient communication in rheumatological disorders. In Newman S, Shipley M (eds) Psychological Aspects of Rheumatic Disease. Baillière's clinical rheumatology. London: Baillière Tindall.

Dargie J, Procter L (1993) Arthritis clinics in practice. Practice Nurse, 1–14 June: 144–8.

Donovan JL, Blake PR, Fleming WG (1989) The patient is not a blank sheet: lay beliefs and their relevance to patient education. British Journal of Rheumatology 28: 58–61.

Feinman J (1997) Fellow travellers. Nursing Times 93 (42): 44–5.

Harris S, Watts N, Jackson R (1993) Four year study of intermittent cyclic etidronate treatment of post menopausal osteoporosis. American Journal of Medicine 95: 557–67.

Havelock M (1998) Audit of compliance of monitoring of slow-acting anti-rheumatic and cytotoxic agents in rheumatology outpatients. Conference presentation, Royal College of Nursing Rheumatology Forum, Bath, March 1998.

Helliwell P (1996) Comparison of a community clinic with a hospital out-patient clinic in rheumatology. British Journal of Rheumatology 35: 385–8.

Helliwell P, O'Hara M (1995) An audit of DMARD monitoring in rheumatoid arthritis. British Journal of Rheumatology 34: 673–5.

Hill J (1997) Patient satisfaction in a nurse led rheumatology clinic. Journal of Advanced Nursing 25 (2): 347–54.

Hopkin SR (1990) Sans awareness. Nursing Times 86 (30): 50–1.

Jones K, Lane D, Holgate S, Price J (1991) A diagnostic and therapeutic challenge. Family Practice 8: 97–9.

Kleerekoper M, Peterson EL, Nelson DA (1991) A randomised trial of sodium fluoride as a treatment for post menopausal osteoporosis. Osteoporosis International 1: 155–61.

Kiel DP, Felson DT, Anderson JJ (1987) Hip fracture and the use of oestrogens in post menopausal women – the framingham study. New England Journal of Medicine 317: 1169–74.

Lindsay R, Aitkin JM, Anderson JB (1976) Long term prevention of postmenopausal osteoporosis by oestrogen. Lancet ii: 1038–41.

Lindsay R, Hart D, Maclean A (1978) Bone response in the termination of oestrogen treatment. Lancet 1: 1325–7.

Mooney J (1996) Audit of rheumatology nurse outreach clinics. Rheumatology in Practice, Winter: 18–20.

Nassen T, Persson I, Adami HO (1990) Hormone replacement therapy and the risk for hip fracture – a prospective population based cohort study. Annals of Internal medicine 13: 95–103.

Recker RR, Karpf DB, Quan H (1995) Three year treatment of osteoporosis with alendronate effects on vertebral fracture incidence. Abstracts of the 77th Annual meeting of the endocrine society, Washington DC.

Reid IR, Ames RW, Evans MC (1993) Effects of calcium supplementation on bone loss in postmenopausal women. New English Journal of Medicine 328: 460–4.

Storm T, Thamsborg G, Steiniche T, Gerrant HK, Sorenson O (1990). Effects of intermittent cyclical etidronate therapy on bone mass and fracture rate in women with postmenopausal osteoporosis. New English Journal of Medicine 322: 1265–71.

Thorne P, Russell R (1973) Diabetic clinics today and tomorrow: mini clinics in general practice. British Medical Journal 2: 534–6.

Walker D (1994) Outreach clinics a consultant replies. Rheumatology Practice 1: 6–8.

Watt NB, Harris ST, Genart H, (1990). Intermittent cyclical etidronate treatment of postmenopausal osteoporosis. New English Journal of Medicine 323: 73–9.

Wolf R (1997) Shared care recording in community care. Nursing Times 93 (28): 52–3.

Index